THE TRUTH ABOUT ADULT SCOLIOSIS

What You Need to Know About History, Treatment Options, and How to Prevent Progression

Also by Dr. Andrew J. Strauss

Your Child Has Scoliosis, Now What Do You Do?
Options to Stay Ahead of the Curve

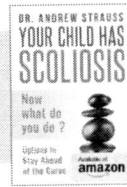

Cover Design by Siniša Poznanović
Typesetting by Eled Černik

Dr. Andrew Jay Strauss
250 West Route 59, Suite 4
Nanuet, New York, 10954
USA

For more information: (845) 624-0010
www.HudsonValleyScoliosis.com

ISBN 978-0-9975789-3-5

Printed in the United States of America

First Edition, April, 2018

Disclaimer

Contents

Acknowledgments

Again, for this, my second book on scoliosis, I give my most deep-hearted thank you to all my patients and their families over the past 36 years of practice. It was my incredible good fortune to find my profession. When I look back on the immense responsibility that so many thousands of parents have entrusted in me, I am truly humbled and driven to continue to increase my skills and knowledge. I am very fortunate to have many colleagues that I consider to be friends in the world of conservative scoliosis care, and I am grateful for their insights and shared passion, which has helped me along my journey as a scoliosis clinician. I apologize for not listing them.

My main sources of support during my working day are my clinical team, our office manager Dawn Rooney, our technical assistants Cinnette Wilder, Laurel Hicks, Darleen Haupt, Alex DeLuca, my associate Dr Richa Desai, and our "builder" Marcus Brownlee. The treatment of scoliosis works best when it is a team approach. Our team is our center's greatest strength. I am fortunate to be surrounded by a group that is dedicated beyond what any team leader could even hope for. I must single out Heather Rooney, our CEO (Chief Experience Officer). Your genuine concern for the practical needs of our patients and their families is only exceeded by your detailed writing assistance and keen editorial vision, which have been essential to the completion of this second major writing project. I know you have once again approached writing this second book as a very personal project and I truly appreciate your commitment to its scientific rigor.

Thank you to my nephew, Tyler Strauss, and Ashton August, founder of YogiApproved.com, for the excellent pictures of Ashton performing yoga postures. My daughters Zaria and Yekira suffered through many days and nights missing their father while he was in his study working on another book; thank you! Thank you to my son, Gabe, who offered enormous practical support and key moments of insight and advice. My wife, Elle, went through a lot and did a lot – I would have given up long ago without her steady support, wisdom, and endless patience. My ultimate gratitude goes to the Holy Blessed One who has orchestrated all.

Prologue. Introduction

What you don't know about adult scoliosis can cause you unnecessary pain. But there *is something you can do.*

Few people realize that options like watching and waiting, pain medications, or even surgery only treat the symptoms of scoliosis, not the real cause. Research on adult scoliosis tells us that a typical adult will experience a progression of their curve, and that the progression will vary from 0.3 to 3.0 degrees per year.

Many adults with scoliosis ultimately discover that their spine is curving too much. That's because one of two things may be happening: Problems they may have **had as a teen** (or younger) have grown worse as they get older, or they are just now starting to develop a gradually worsening curvature of their spine that they may have **never had as a teen**.

Many find that the only scoliosis treatment options presented to them as an adult are the traditional ones, and they are not very satisfying. Their scoliosis leaves them feeling hopeless. They feel like their curve's slow but relentless progression is out of control. They worry about how their condition will progress and worsen over time.

If you are one of these people, I have great news for you:

Your condition is treatable. There is hope.

The 4 Most Dangerous Scoliosis Myths

These myths cause unnecessary pain, disability, and further progression of your curves.

When scoliosis patients believe these myths, they are prevented from seeking a solution for their scoliosis *before* pain and disability start to develop. Here are some of the most prevalent myths about adult scoliosis that cause patients to suffer more than they need to.

Myth #1: Mild scoliosis curves rarely progress after skeletal maturity

Many scoliosis patients have heard again and again that their condition is unlikely to deteriorate as they get older, especially if their curve is mild. But more recent and advanced studies have shown this just isn't true. There are different kinds of scoliosis and some of them are likely to result in a greater, less-predictable progression of the curve over the course of your life. No matter what kind of scoliosis you have, your curve is most likely to continue to worsen later in life.

Even if your scoliosis began during adolescence and you've seen little increase in your curve over time, you will learn that many adult scoliosis sufferers have seen drastic increases in their curve angle later in life. Even a small yearly progression of 0.3 degrees per year adds up over a lifetime!

Myth #2: Curves always progress predictably

If it's been a while since you were first diagnosed with scoliosis, you may be under the impression that your curve will progress at the same rate that it always has. This is not always true. While the type of scoliosis you have is a factor, many patients experience more drastic and unpredictable progression of their curves later in life.

Myth #3: If you have no pain from scoliosis now, you never will

In the chapters that follow, I will show you the research findings and patient testimonials that demonstrate how pain is very likely to develop later in life

— even if you had no pain from your scoliosis as an adolescent or young adult. In fact, one study indicated that **92% of adult scoliosis sufferers reported pain from their scoliosis.**

Myth #4: There is nothing you can do, short of a major spinal surgery involving rods and fusion of the spinal bones

One of the saddest and most destructive myths of all is perpetuated by medical professionals and specialists themselves. If you have scoliosis, there's no doubt that you've heard this before:

> *"There is nothing you can do to change the progression of your curve. You can only 'watch and wait.'" Take over the counter pain medicine, have some physical therapy, and when it gets bad enough, return and we will perform surgery."*

Here's the Truth:

Even mild curves of less than 30 degrees have a greater chance of getting worse during later adulthood than they did during your 20s or 30s, and some scoliosis sufferers are at even higher risk than others. This is due to spinal degeneration that may accompany the aging process.

Curves do not always progress predictably, and elderly scoliosis sufferers are more likely than any other adult age group to experience unpredictable, rapid progression of their curves. This is especially true for the type of adult scoliosis that starts later in life.

Even if you've never experienced pain from your scoliosis, there is a greater chance of pain developing because of your scoliosis later in life. This is true even if you have a mild curve now.

Much of the pain and deterioration of adult scoliosis is preventable

In this book, you will learn:

- Why much of what you've been told about your scoliosis condition is completely wrong.

- What risk factors can contribute to the onset of pain and disability later in your life, even if you've never experienced pain or disability from your scoliosis before.

- How menopause is known to be a time of accelerating scoliosis progression and increased pain.

- How to prevent the rapid deterioration of your curves as you age.

- How to reduce or eliminate pain from scoliosis without risky surgery or reliance on pain medicine. You will also learn about how modern and innovative braces are proven to help adult scoliosis patients.

- What you can do *starting right now* to improve your quality of life and have a brighter future.

The 4 Biggest Concerns for Adult Scoliosis Sufferers

There is a big difference between adolescent scoliosis and adult scoliosis. If you've had scoliosis for a long time, you may wrongly believe that your condition will be no different in the future than it has been up to this point in your life.

Adult scoliosis patients have two main concerns that don't apply to a majority of adolescent sufferers. They are:

- Pain

- Disability

Adult and adolescent scoliosis share two other main concerns:

- Progression

- Aesthetics

Each of these concerns can contribute to the deterioration of a scoliosis patient's quality of life as they get older.

Pain

Though it is rare for scoliosis to cause pain in adolescence, pain is a common symptom of adult scoliosis. The patients in my office receiving adult scoliosis treatment often say the same thing. They were told they had scoliosis as a child or teen and were advised to "watch and wait." Then, around middle age, quite often sooner, they begin to experience back pain, hip pain, or other symptoms only to discover that scoliosis is the underlying culprit.

Disability

Another terrible consequence of untreated scoliosis is disability. You lose your freedom to do the things that you love to do and become less and less independent. Some severe scoliosis sufferers cannot even stand or walk because their condition is so degenerative. This is known as postural collapse and occurs in adults due to the relentless effect of gravity on the scoliotic spine.

As scoliosis patients become older, the likelihood of disability increases. Without treatment, disability from very large scoliosis can cause you to become extremely limited in your activities, unable to perform your normal duties without assistance, and completely without the freedom to do the things that you enjoy.

Progression

Even worse than the severe pain or limiting disability that can occur for scoliosis sufferers is the feeling of utter helplessness to do anything about it. When you do not receive treatment for scoliosis and simply "watch and wait," you are vulnerable to the likely outcome that your curve will get much worse over time.

Research shows that the curve progression in an adult will vary between 0.3 to 3.0 degrees per year, depending on the shape of the curve, overall curve size, and the age of the scoliosis onset.

It was previously thought that progression only happens for people with more extreme curves of more than 30 or 40 degrees. But more recent studies have proven that certain scoliosis curves can and *often do progress drastically and in a shorter period of time, especially as you get older.*

No one can say definitively how your curves will progress.

There is no telling how your curve will progress in the future, no matter what doctors predict based on other patients. The truth is that no one can tell the future. That's why it is so important to get effective treatment for your scoliosis instead of waiting, only to find that you are one of those unlucky scoliosis patients whose curve progressed.

Aesthetics

While pain, disability, and the progression of your curves are the most serious and urgent results of adult scoliosis, the way you look when you go about your daily life is a very real and important consideration for scoliosis sufferers.

In addition to worrying about the possibility of your condition deteriorating over time and resulting in pain, you may sometimes feel self-conscious because of the way your scoliosis makes you look.

So many scoliosis sufferers can relate to this feeling of being different from everyone else. Even if you are experiencing no pain, your scoliosis appears as a disability in the eyes of people you see at work, at the supermarket, in interviews, at gatherings with friends, and everywhere you go.

The good news is that treatment for your scoliosis can stabilise, and typically even modestly reduce, your scoliosis and allow you to experience less pain, disability, progression, and self-consciousness. **Research shows that even if the curve can only be modestly reduced, significant postural improvement is still very possible!**

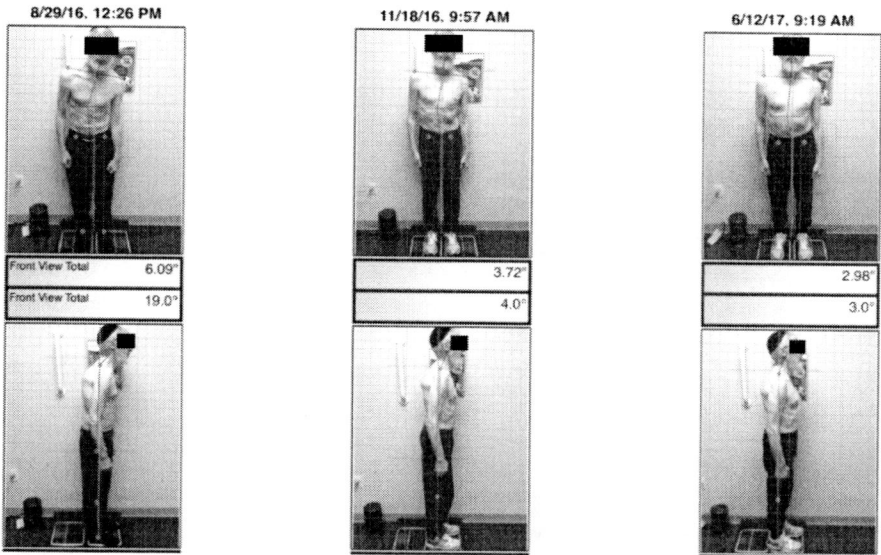

8/29/16. 12:26 PM   11/18/16. 9:57 AM   6/12/17. 9:19 AM

| Front View Total | 6.09° |
| Front View Total | 19.0° |

| | 3.72° |
| | 4.0° |

| | 2.98° |
| | 3.0° |

The Traditional Options — None Satisfactory

Below are what you've been told by most orthodox medical authorities are your only options to experience relief from your scoliosis. As you will see, none of them is satisfactory because they do not address the root cause of scoliosis. Additionally, they are risky, uncertain, and in some cases, downright dangerous.

Bad Option #1: "Watch and Wait:"
Observe the Scoliosis and Do Nothing

Sadly, it is common practice for doctors to recommend "observing" mild, moderate, (and even sometimes severe) scoliosis curves, also called a "watch-and-wait" approach. What this really boils down to is that, once the scoliosis is discovered, it is re-x-rayed (in adults this will usually be annually) until it progresses past a 50-60 degree curve. Then, the "observing" doctor states that the patient is a candidate for spinal surgery. (*I devote 6 chapters in this book to surgery, explaining why it should be seen only as a last-resort treatment choice.*)

As I have said and will elaborate on in this book, it is risky, dangerous, and uncertain to take this traditional advice of "watch and wait." It is possible for treatment to prevent further progression and pain, but it is more challenging to treat progression and pain once it has already begun.

Besides this, watch-and-wait has serious implications for your mental health. Traditional medicine does not always account for the fear, uncertainty, and hopelessness that is a part of the daily lives of those who suffer with scoliosis.

Bluntly, "watch and wait" is not a scoliosis treatment; it is just doing nothing and hoping the scoliosis won't get worse. It will.

> *Many times, I have had patients come into my practice saying, "It was just a mild scoliosis curve until suddenly it just took off and progressed to over 50 degrees. Now my doctor is recommending spinal fusion surgery!"*

Bad Option #2: Risky and Dangerous Surgery

Nearly every scoliosis sufferer has considered the option of surgery as a solution. Many patients who feel helpless to improve their condition think that this is the only way they can have control over their situation. It's easy to see why: faced with daily pain and disability, the patient would rather pursue the small chance of hope that surgery will help them than continue with what they *know* will happen if they watch and wait — exactly the prison they have experienced so far, along with the chance that their condition will get even worse over time.

Most orthopedic specialists try very hard to avoid performing surgery for scoliosis in adults. It is a complex procedure prone to complications.

Surgery to correct scoliosis involves placing a metal rod or cage along the spine in an effort to prevent further curvature. The surgeon uses screws and bone grafts to keep the rod or cage in place next to the spine. This is called "fusion surgery." The spinal bones are fused together, destroying the joints of the spine.

The surgeon will create a long, deep incision along the spine and will spread the ribs if he needs to access the middle section of the spine. This leaves a conspicuous scar and involves a lengthy and painful recovery period.

High risk of complication: According to a 2002 German study on the long-term effects of surgery on idiopathic scoliosis, "40 percent of operated patients with idiopathic scoliosis were legally defined as severely handicapped persons" after having rod and fusion surgery.

Bad Option #3: Treat Only the Pain.

Popping pills is a dead-end treatment because the underlying issue is never addressed, the pills will eventually lead to other possibly serious health complications, and your scoliosis will likely continue to worsen over time....

Solutions Do Exist

This book is a natural outgrowth of my mission to serve scoliosis patients by educating them and their families about the treatment alternatives available to them.

My hope is that, by reading this book and educating yourself about scoliosis, you'll be able to make informed choices about the best treatment option for you. You also will be able to determine which type of care you should accept first, and which treatment options should be your last resort in almost any scenario.

About Me

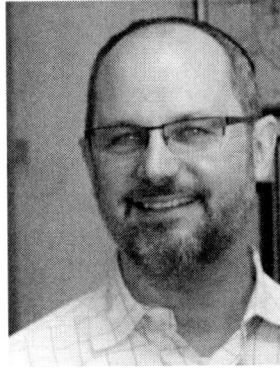

Dr. Andrew Strauss, BS, MS, DC

My journey to become a chiropractic doctor started with my own personal experience of chiropractic's healing power as a young boy. In my youth, my health was destroyed by irregular but severe chest pains. My family consulted traditional medical specialists, but nothing relieved my excruciating discomfort. I was told there was nothing to be done, just "live with it."

It wasn't until my family ignored traditional medicine and tried chiropractic care in my teens that I experienced a phenomenal cure for this debilitating pain. At that point, I made the decision to devote my life to providing the health-restoring healing art of chiropractic.

I graduated with a Bachelor of Science in Biology with honors from the University of New Hampshire in 1978. I went on to study chiropractic at Palmer College of Chiropractic in Davenport, Iowa, the world's oldest and largest chiropractic college. I graduated with honors in 1982.

I have a Master of Applied Science degree in acupuncture from the Royal Melbourne Institute of Technology, a Doctorate in Traditional Medicines from Medicina Alternativa, and a graduate diploma in Chinese herbalism. Other post-graduate training has included advanced studies in spinal mechanics, ISICO World Masters of Scoliosis, scoliosis-specific exercise training and clinical nutrition, as well as courses in various physical therapies and diagnostics such as computerized spinal decompression, whole-body vibration, foot orthotics, manipulation under anesthesia, laser acupuncture, 3D scoliosis bracing design, electromyography and radiology.

All of this paved the way for my work in the field of scoliosis treatment, a vocation that has now spanned 36 years. After studying spinal biomechanics with Dr. Dennis Woggon in the early 1980s, I continued working closely with him and the CLEAR Scoliosis Institute to gain its highest level of certification. I am the vice president of CLEAR, a nonprofit scoliosis institution for which I lecture and serve on the technique advisory committee. I am a member of the Palmer College of Chiropractic Alumni Association, past president of the Upper Cervical Society, member The International Chiropractic Pediatric Association and member of the American Academy of Spine Physicians. I am also a member of and lecturer for the International Chiropractors Association.

On a personal note, I am married to Elle, and we have two daughters and a son.

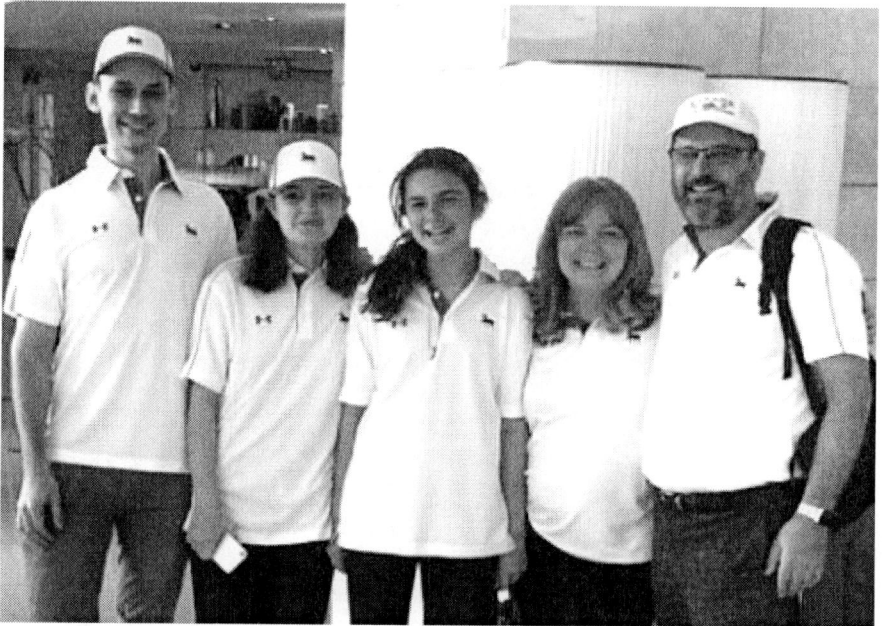

About My Treatment Program

In my work, I've seen the physical and emotional trauma caused by scoliosis and have made it my mission to treat and reduce scoliosis cases. In most instances, I have been able to accomplish this without the use of braces or sending patients to surgery. My practice, the Hudson Valley Scoliosis Correction Center just outside New York City, offers conservative and natural healing focused on the treatment of scoliosis.

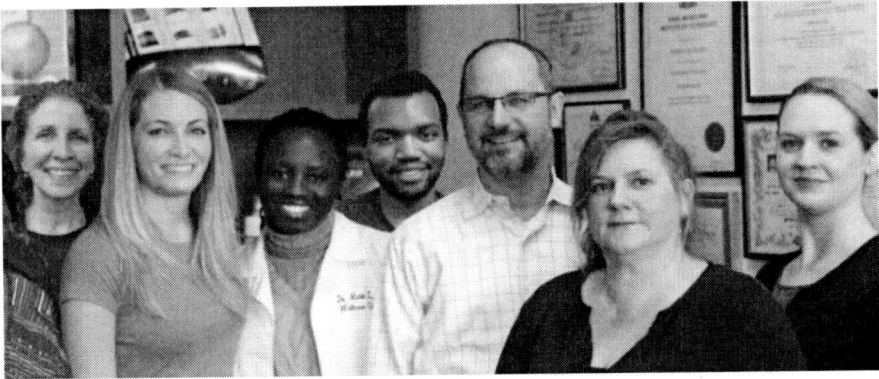

My team and I utilize a wide variety of chiropractic techniques — an American science more than 100 years old — modern applications of Chinese medicine, which dates back 3,000 years; and clinical nutrition and wellness practices, which have stood the test of time.

Combined with a wide knowledge and application of the latest physical therapeutic and orthotic tools as well as scoliosis-specific exercise-based treatment strategies from all over the world, our center is providing dramatic help for scoliosis sufferers.

These newer techniques work well because they target the root cause of scoliosis rather than just the symptoms. By seeking to maximize the natural strengths of the body and its capacity to heal itself, I am able to help patients help themselves. The basic principle guiding our center is to empower patients to help themselves by developing for them a custom-designed home exercise program. We teach the person how to help themselves.

Scoliosis can be a very scary and traumatic condition.

However, this book's purpose is not meant to make you anxious. It's meant to calm the minds of patients and their families. Scoliosis is the subject of much research, and knowledge is power!

You could go from specialist to specialist seeking opinions without ever knowing that there is an alternative treatment for the condition, one shown to be effective in stabilizing and typically even reducing scoliosis curves and minimizing – even eliminating – pain by addressing the *CAUSE* of scoliosis.

I invite you on a journey of education and discovery. The greatest way to eliminate any fear you may have about your scoliosis is to become educated about scoliosis in general.

As you read through this book, keep in mind that this book is written for Adult Scoliosis patients… this means those patients who have passed skeletal maturity. In females, this means patients who are approximately 16-18 and older; in males, 17-19 and older. The age of skeletal maturity varies from person to person.

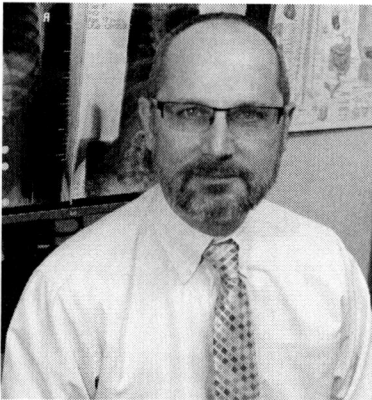

Yours in health,

Dr. Andrew Strauss, BS, DC, MS

P.S. Remember that all severe scoliosis curves have one thing in common; they started out as mild curves and progressively got worse. Do something about your child's scoliosis N-O-W and reclaim control over your family's life.

I. ADULT SCOLIOSIS – WHAT YOU NEED TO KNOW

Chapter 1. The World of Scoliosis: Definitions and Diagnosis

Hippocrates, the ancient Greek physician, first wrote of spine deformity in 460 B.C. Approximately five centuries later, the Greek physician Galen introduced specific terms for normal and abnormal spinal curves. He coined medical terms such as **"scoliosis," "kyphosis"** and **"lordosis."** The word "scoliosis" comes from a Greek word meaning "crooked." So essentially, scoliosis means "crooked back" or "crooked spine." The healthy spine has normal curves when looking from the side, but it should appear straight when looking from behind.

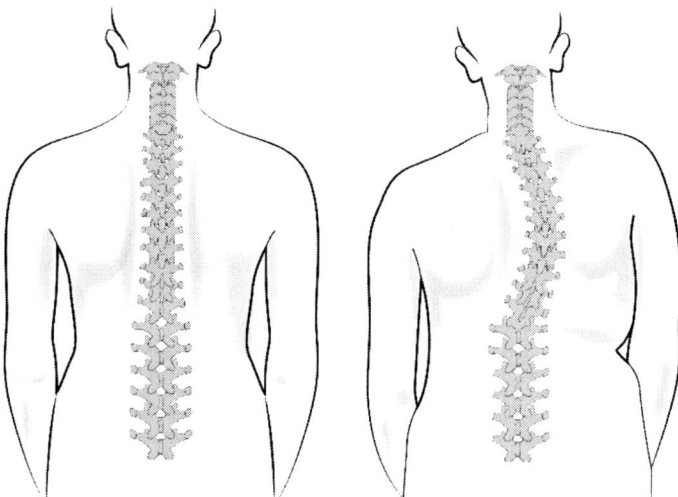

Normal Spine   Scoliosis

Scoliosis is a term used to describe a spine that has twisted abnormally to the side. Kyphosis is a curve seen from the side in which the spine is bent forward. There is a normal kyphosis in the mid back, or thoracic spine region. Lordosis is a curve seen from the side in which the spine is bent backward. There is normal lordosis in the cervical spine and the lumbar spine.

People with scoliosis develop one or more additional curves to the sides, and the bones of the spine twist on each other, forming C-shaped or S-shaped curvatures. It may or may not be noticeable to others.

Two Main Types of Adult Scoliosis[1]:

Adolescent Idiopathic Scoliosis in Adults (ASA): Idiopathic scoliosis from childhood that has progressed into adulthood. This "teenage scoliosis" will combine with degenerative changes (deterioration) to the spine as the patient ages. The increasing curve size and arthritis of the spinal joints (that are being stressed by an imbalanced spine) begin to provoke the pain that compels the patient to seek treatment. Idiopathic means "no known cause," and idiopathic scoliosis is the most common type of childhood scoliosis (96 percent) sometimes occurring as early as the age of first walking (infantile scoliosis), but more typically around 10 years of age.

De Novo, also known as Degenerative Scoliosis (DS): A scoliosis occurring in individuals whose bones have fully developed, typically in middle age or older. This type of scoliosis results from imbalanced degeneration of the spinal discs and is often accompanied by spinal stenosis (narrowing of the spaces within the spine). It is most often found in the thoracolumbar (mid to lower back) or lumbar (lower back) regions of the spine. It may be preceded by a minor scoliosis in the teen years, or it may spontaneously develop in a spine that has had no scoliosis previously.

Structural Scoliosis in Adults: The spine has a structural problem caused by something from outside the spine. The cause could be a variety of neurologically-based or muscle-based diseases; injuries to the spine, legs or pelvis;

---

1 Smith JS, Shaffrey CI, Kuntz CT et al. Classification systems for adolescent and adult scoliosis. *Neurosugery.* 2008;63 (3 Suppl):16-24.

infection of the bones; a result of birth defects; some causes of a short leg; or pelvic unbalancing.

Metabolic bone disease: This type of scoliosis in adults is due to the effects of a metabolic bone disease leading to fracture. It is often found in combination with imbalanced disc degeneration. The most common metabolic disease associated with scoliosis in adults is osteoporosis.

Non-structural Scoliosis (also called "functional scoliosis"): The spine is structurally normal, and the curve is temporary. A typical cause for this type of scoliosis is muscle spasm causing temporary postural changes.

In some cases of a mild adolescent idiopathic scoliosis that worsens later in adulthood, it can be difficult to classify the scoliosis!

Without a patient's history, it is difficult to determine the age that the patient first began to develop scoliosis.

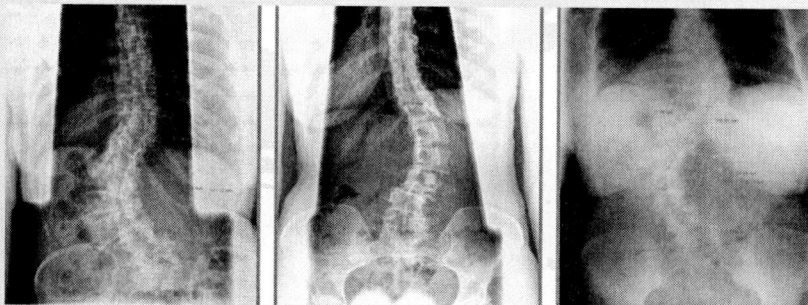

The above images display the variety of adult scoliosis presentations.

Why Do People Get Scoliosis?

If we remove cases of obvious trauma, disease, or congenital causes, scoliosis **"etiology"** (study of a condition's cause) holds mostly unanswered questions when dealing with the type of scoliosis that develops in childhood. In most people, there is no universally accepted reason for the development of "teen scoliosis." While the exact mechanism of the development of de novo scoliosis in adults has yet to be fully clarified, age-related degeneration of the spine is the most common underlying cause. The natural "normal" curves of the spine play an important role in degenerative changes and the pain of adult scoliosis (see illustration in Ch 2, p. 22). When these "normal" curves are reduced or absent, adult scoliosis becomes more common.

Small curve idiopathic scoliosis of childhood is equally common in girls and boys. Larger curves are much more common in girls than boys. It can be seen at any age, but it is typically first noticed in those older than 10 years of age. About four out of every 100 children have some form of scoliosis. The percentage of adults with adolescent idiopathic scoliosis becomes much much larger. Remember that all the children with idiopathic scoliosis eventually become adults with scoliosis!

The percentage of people with adult degenerative scoliosis also increases with age. De novo or adult degenerative scoliosis is considered a disease of aging. Studies have reported the prevalence of all types of scoliosis in adults to be up to 68 percent.[2]

Teen scoliosis can run in families, and modern theories suggest a genetic link. An adult who has had scoliosis from childhood should see that their children or grandchildren are screened regularly for scoliosis. Physicians use medical and family history and a physical exam when checking a person for scoliosis. An x-ray of the spine will confirm if a person has scoliosis. The scoliosis x-ray lets the doctor measure the angle of the curve in degrees and see its location, shape and pattern.

Is Scoliosis Painful?

In the large majority of cases, scoliotic curves in children will not cause pain. However, pain is the most common reason for adults to seek care for their scoliosis. In an adult patient, if the curve is less than 30 degrees, it may or may not increase in size before the age of 50 but may increase after that age

---

2 Kotwal S, Pumberger M, Hughes A, et al. Degenerative Scoliosis: a review. HSS J. 2011;7(3): 257-64

due to the combination of scoliosis and degenerative changes to the spine. If the curve is greater than 30 degrees, it is highly likely to increase in size over the person's life, with pain developing between 30 and 50 years of age and beyond. If there is pain present, treatment should always be designed to alleviate pain first, then stop curve progression and stabilize the curve corrections. In many cases a modest reduction in curve size is possible.

All large scoliosis curves have one thing in common; they started as small curves! It is much easier to treat a smaller-sized scoliosis and effectively reduce the curve, preventing curve progression and the associated pain and disability. If you or a family member have a smaller curve, get it corrected before it has a chance to develop into a larger curve. Why watch and wait until it becomes larger?

> To such an extent does nature delight and abound in variety that among her trees there is not one plant to be found which is exactly like another; and not only among the plants, but among the boughs, the leaves and the fruits, you will not find one which is exactly similar to another.
>
> **– Leonardo da Vinci**

Chapter 2. The Many Forms of Scoliosis

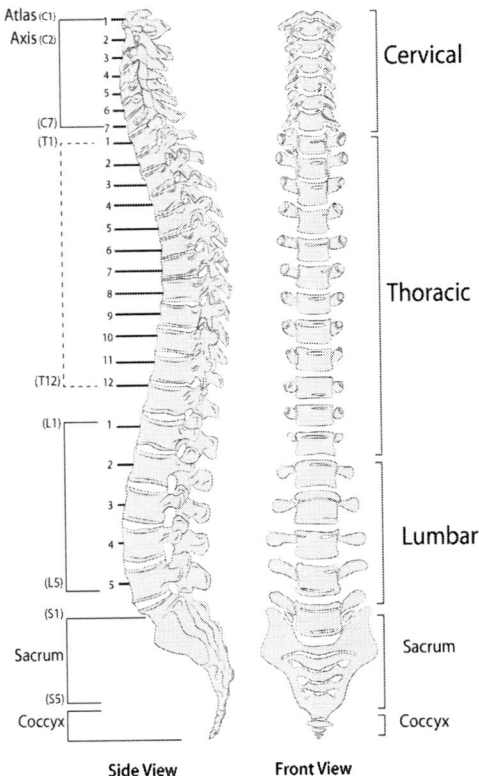

Atlas (C1)
Axis (C2)

(C7)
(T1)

(T12)

(L1)

(L5)
(S1)
Sacrum
(S5)
Coccyx

Side View   **Front View**

Cervical

Thoracic

Lumbar

Sacrum

Coccyx

Scoliosis is not one specific disease, but rather the word is a term used to describe any abnormal, sideways or **lateral curvature** of the spine. Viewed from the back, a typical spine looks straight. If the spine curves, it can show up as a curve to either side. It can be a single curve shaped like the letter C — or **"C-shaped scoliosis"** — or the spine can have two curves, resembling the letter S — or **"S-shaped scoliosis."** In rare cases, the spine contorts into triple or quadruple curves.

The spine has 24 vertebrae that are divided into three sections: **cervical** (the seven vertebrae of the neck), **thoracic** (the 12 vertebrae of the middle back), and **lumbar** (the five vertebrae of the lower back).

Scoliosis can occur in the neck **(cervical spine scoliosis)**, in the middle back **(thoracic spine scoliosis)** and in the lower back **(lumbar spine scoliosis)**. Scoliosis can mix the areas of the spine involved in the curve in various combinations.

For example, a **lumbar scoliosis** (the most common form seen in adult degenerative scoliosis) typically involves a curve to the left in the lower back that affects an average of five vertebrae. **Thoracolumbar scoliosis** is curvature that includes vertebrae in both the lower thoracic and upper lumbar portions of the spine. Scoliosis that involves both the thoracic and lumbar spinal regions are called **"double major curves"**.

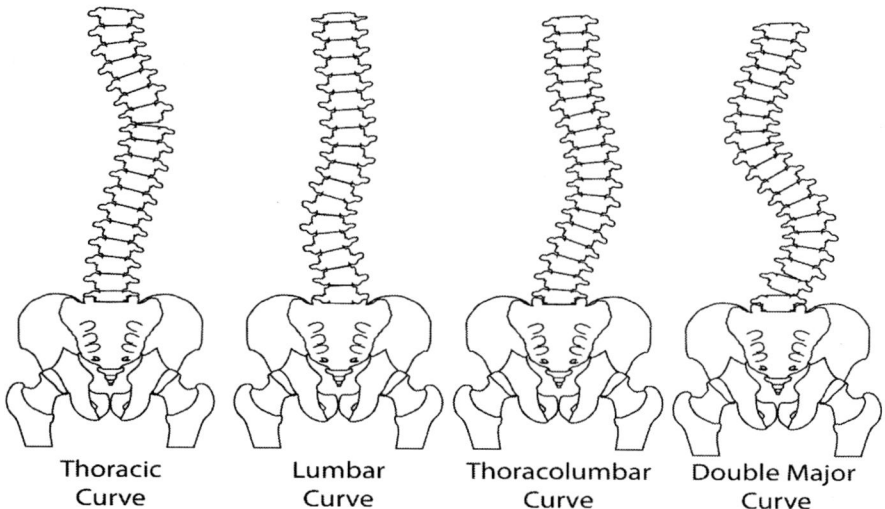

| Thoracic Curve | Lumbar Curve | Thoracolumbar Curve | Double Major Curve |

Common Scoliosis Terms Explained

Dextroscoliosis is a spinal curve to the right ("dextro" means right). Usually occurring in the thoracic spine, this is the most common type of curve. It can occur on its own (forming a C-curve) or with another curve bending the opposite way in the lower spine (forming an S-curve). The reason a right-

hand or "dextro" thoracic scoliosis is most common is that the body naturally avoids the heart which is located to the left of the midline of the torso.

Levoscoliosis is a spinal curve to the left ("levo" means left). Common in
the lumbar spine, the rare occurrence of levoscoliosis in the thoracic spine
indicates a higher probability that the scoliosis may be secondary to a some
kind of disease or illness such as a spinal cord tumor (Syrinx), spinal cord
tethering, or Chiari syndrome.[3] Chiari means the cerebellum is entering the
spine instead of staying in the skull. In the case of a levoscoliosis in the
thoracic spine, an MRI study often is recommended. Adults with de novo
scoliosis most commonly present with a levoscoliosis in the lumbar spine.

Kyphosis is a forward-bending curve of the spine, when seen from the side.
There is a normal kyphosis in the middle (thoracic) spine, but if the spine is
bent excessively forward, it is classified as a **kyphotic spine**. This may sound
confusing, but when the thoracic spine is referred to as kyphotic on a report,
that is always due to excessive kyphosis as there would be no reference to
this with normal findings.

Kyphoscoliosis is an abnormal curvature of the spine consisting of *both*
kyphosis and scoliosis. This is a common finding in adult de novo scoliosis.

Lordosis is a curve that — when seen from the side — features a spine bent
posteriorly or backward in the cervical neck region or the lower back/lum-
bar area. Both excessively large or excessively small amounts of lordosis can
be a problem.

How Can the Most Common Type of Scoliosis Have No Known Cause?

The type of structural scoliosis that has no known cause occurs in approximately 4 percent of children. Research shows adolescent idiopathic scoliosis
(AIS) affects 1-3 percent of children in the at-risk population of 10-16 years

---

3 "Chiari Malformation Fact Sheet." 2006. 23 Mar. 2016 http://www.ninds.nih.gov/
disorders/chiari/detail_chiari.htm

age.[4] When we add in children younger than 10, we arrive at the figure of 4 percent. If we include adult numbers in our calculations, the incidence percentage is much higher.

> *Think about it.… If all the children that have adolescent idiopathic scoliosis grow up to be adults with adolescent scoliosis, the percentage of those afflicted gets very large.*

As mentioned previously, the term "idiopathic" means a condition or disease with no known cause. Idiopathic scoliosis is by far the most common cause of scoliosis. Vast amounts of research have been done over many years to determine what causes it, but at the time of this writing there is no definitive answer. Many theories have been put forward. Yes, most scientists will agree that there is a genetic connection, but what triggers the expression of these weakened genes is still a puzzle. Don't be surprised; there are many conditions that are not fully understood.

Medical science is making steady progress on figuring scoliosis out. Risk factors that are linked to triggering the genetic expression of scoliosis present themselves in many forms. The technical word for this is "epigenetics." Some of the possible factors include: trauma to the spine, exposure to certain bacteria types, hormonal imbalances, poor posture, or even nutritional deficiencies.

> *Idiopathic scoliosis rarely causes pain during childhood but is often painful during one's later years. Once scoliosis is detected (in either the child or the adult), it should be closely monitored by a scoliosis professional who will initiate a proactive plan to ensure the curve does not progress and — if possible — will be reduced and stabilized. Active custom-designed exercise therapy prescribed by a scoliosis expert is currently recognized as the best starting point for both mild to moderate curves in a child as well as for adults wanting to avoid surgery.*

---

4 Weinstein, S.L. "PubMed – NCBI." 2008. 26 Apr. 2016
http://www.ncbi.nlm.nih.gov/pubmed/18456103

To More Fully Understand Scoliosis, Let's Look at the 4 Types of Idiopathic Scoliosis

Idiopathic scoliosis has been somewhat artificially divided into four sub-groups according to age: **infantile** (0-3 years), **juvenile** (4-10 years), and **adolescent** (11- maturity). Once maturity is reached, idiopathic scoliosis is classified as **adolescent scoliosis in an adult (ASA).**

Please keep in mind that if the scoliosis started in a 12-year-old, but was not identified (diagnosed) until adulthood, it could still be referred to mistakenly as "adult onset scoliosis." In some cases, it can be difficult or impossible to determine the age period when the scoliosis originally formed. This is a big problem when attempting to make sense of the development of scoliosis. But, let's still take a look at this classification system anyway.

Infantile Idiopathic Scoliosis – Yes, Babies Can Have Scoliosis!

Infantile scoliosis is defined as scoliosis that is first diagnosed in a child between birth and 3 years of age. Ninety percent of early onset scoliosis will resolve without treatment.[5]

Those that do not resolve can be difficult to manage. Frequent check-ups are needed, and if progression is seen, aggressive non-surgical treatment must be started. The child will not be able to benefit from an exercise-based program at this age. The best forms of care start with either serial plaster casting or the use of hard plastic bracing methods. There are currently a variety of invasive surgical methods based on the insertion of expandable rods used for treating infantile scoliosis.

Juvenile Idiopathic Scoliosis: Age 4-10

Juvenile onset scoliosis is defined as spinal curves diagnosed between ages 3–10. It is less common than adolescent scoliosis, but still makes up about

---

5 "Infantile Scoliosis – Medscape Reference." 23 Mar. 2016 http://emedicine.medscape.com/article/1259899-overview

10–15 percent of all scoliosis cases.[6] I have found children over the age of seven can benefit from exercise-based care programs. Success rates in younger children are high with proper coaching from a dedicated doctor and his staff AND when combined with the help of a well-trained parent, guardian or even a school teacher. A team approach works best.

Adolescent Idiopathic Scoliosis: Tweens and Teens

Adolescent idiopathic scoliosis (AIS) occurs in children ages 11–18 years and comprises approximately 80 percent of all cases of idiopathic scoliosis diagnosed during childhood. This age range is when rapid growth typically occurs, which is why a curve at this stage should be monitored closely as the child's skeleton develops. This is the age of highest risk of progression. Patients are very motivated to perform the home-exercise routines to avoid bracing and surgery. Adolescents are old enough to understand the choices they are making and typically want surgery ONLY as a last resort!

Adolescent Scoliosis in an Adult

Once skeletal maturity is reached, a patient with adolescent idiopathic scoliosis is now referred to as having adolescent scoliosis in an adult (ASA). A patient with ASA will benefit greatly from treatment for pain control, cosmetic improvement, slowing or stopping progression, and in many cases, some curve reduction. Pain unfortunately is the dominant reason adults with scoliosis seek treatment. Normal degenerative changes of the spine may be accelerated by the scoliosis curvature and the patient may be at higher risk for skeletal pain or extremity pain due to nerve compression.

Yes, Adults Can Develop Scoliosis, Too!

Not to be confused with adolescent scoliosis in an adult (ASA), **adult scoliosis also known as adult onset scoliosis or de novo scoliosis** is most typically a degenerative scoliosis, which is a side-to-side curvature of the spine associated with degeneration of the spinal joints. Degenerative scoliosis

6 Wick, JM. "Infantile and Juvenile Scoliosis: The Crooked Path to ..." 2009. 25 Apr. 2016 http://www.aornjournal.org/article/S0001-2092(09)00551-1/abstract

shows up in middle-aged and older adults, most frequently in people aged 35–65. Typically, a C-shaped curve forms in the lumbar spine. It can occur due to wear and tear causing osteoarthritis in the spine, or "spondylosis." Age related weakening of the normal ligaments and other soft tissues of the spine combined with abnormal bone spurs can lead to significant spinal slippage and twisting. This can result in an abnormal curvature of the spine.

The spine can also be affected by osteoporosis, vertebral compression fractures, and disc degeneration. These changes and their associated pain cause the body to lean to one side in an effort to reduce the postural strains causing spinal deformity.

Degenerative scoliosis is the most common form of scoliosis in adults and is often seen in those who had a milder form of scoliosis as a child.

> **Who is most likely to get scoliosis?** *Age is a primary underlying risk factor with an increased prevalence of scoliosis as adults age. Prevalence rates differed among races (e.g., adult scoliosis is nearly twice as common for Caucasians as for African Americans) but similar for men and women. There is no difference in the distribution of curve severity by gender or age, and African Americans are much more likely to have mild curves than other races.*

Types of Scoliosis for Which We Know the Cause

Structural scoliosis presents as a fixed curve and is treated case by case. It can be caused by a variety of neurological and/or muscular disorders or birth defects such as hemivertebra, in which one side of a vertebra fails to form normally before birth. The vertebrae can fail to form completely or fail to separate from each other during fetal development. This type of scoliosis also can result from significant leg length discrepancies, metabolic diseases, connective tissue disorders, rheumatic disease, or injury to the spine, legs or pelvis.

The underlying cause of most structural scoliosis stems from unknown factors and is not related to any physical problems (this type of structural scoliosis is referred to as idiopathic scoliosis – no known cause).

Structural scoliosis develops in people with other disorders, (i.e. birth defects, muscular dystrophy, cerebral palsy, or Marfan's disease). People with these conditions often develop a long C-curve. Their muscles are just not able to hold their spines straight.

Non-structural (functional) scoliosis: Non-structural scoliosis is a curve in the spine without rotation. It is reversible because it is caused by a treatable condition such as pain or muscle spasm. In this type of scoliosis, the spinal curvature is a healthy adaptation to a temporary problem.[7]

Compensatory scoliosis: This spinal curve disappears when the patient sits. It may be caused by either a short leg, misshaped pelvic bones, or a pelvic tilt due to hip contracture. This type of curve will straighten significantly with side-bending to produce spinal balance. Compensatory scoliosis can be caused by a misalignment of the spine ("vertebral subluxation" or "pinched nerve"). When mild, this type of scoliosis can be treated with great success by a general practice chiropractor.

The age of onset combined with the current age of the patient and the location of the scoliosis determines the classification of the scoliosis. For example, a 30-year-old with an adolescent onset structural curve of unknown cause in the thoracic spine is called "thoracic adolescent idiopathic scoliosis in an adult." The exact definition of the curve has implications for determining scoliosis progression and scoliosis treatment.

This is an explanation of a few basic terms used to classify scoliosis. If it appears complicated, it is. Don't make the mistake of assuming you have enough understanding to self-diagnose. There are even more complicated classifications for scoliosis such as the Rigo, King and Lenke classification systems.[8]

It's always best to consult your physician who has expertise in scoliosis with any questions you may have about your scoliosis diagnosis.

---

7 Kotwal S, Pumberger M, Hughes A, et al. Degenerative Scoliosis: a review. HSS J. 2011;7(3): 257-64

8 "Lenke Classification System for Scoliosis | Lawrence Lenke ..." 2012. 24 Mar. 2016. http://spinal-deformity-surgeon.com/a-leader-in-spinal-deformity/lenke-classification-system-for-scoliosis/

Chapter 3. How to Tell if You Have Scoliosis

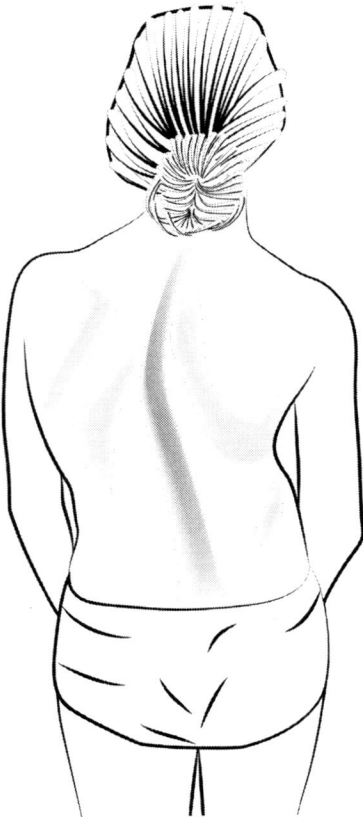

Often, scoliosis is first noticed by a friend or family member. Since changes in the spine happen gradually and always begin as a smaller curve, it may go unnoticed by the individual. As the curve becomes more severe, individuals will begin to notice that their clothes do not fit the same or that pant legs are shorter on one side than the other. Perhaps a friend notices that you're walking with one hip more prominent than the other.

The most common sign of scoliosis is an abnormal shape of the torso. While a healthy spine has a natural curvature when viewed from the side, it appears as a straight line when viewed from the back. However, an individual with a significant scoliosis will appear to have a side-to-side curve in their spine when viewed from behind.

What to Look Out For

Scoliosis may cause the head to appear off center or one hip or shoulder to be higher on one side of the body. You may have a more obvious curve or prominence on one side of the rib cage from the twisting of the vertebrae and ribs.

If scoliosis sufferers bend forward to touch their toes, thoracic curves will make one shoulder blade stick out prominently. Curves in the lumbar region of the back will show very little evidence of their existence when bending forward. It is the imbalance in the waist that is the telling sign. If the scoliosis is very severe, it can make it difficult for the heart and lungs to work properly. This can cause shortness of breath and chest pain.

When back pain is present with scoliosis, it may be because the curve in the spine is causing stress and pressure on the spinal discs, nerves, muscles, ligaments or joints. Combine this with degeneration (also known as arthritis) of the spinal joints and you can understand why there can be significant pain and disability. Whether you have back pain associated with scoliosis or not, it is very important that you see a doctor to find out what is causing any pains you may be experiencing.

Signs of Scoliosis in the Adult

Even without an x-ray of the spine, there are several common physical signs that may indicate scoliosis. It is not uncommon for it to be discovered during a routine physical exam when your physician does a full body scan looking for skin lesions.

Scoliosis Curve Patterns

Right Thoracic
Curver of 70°

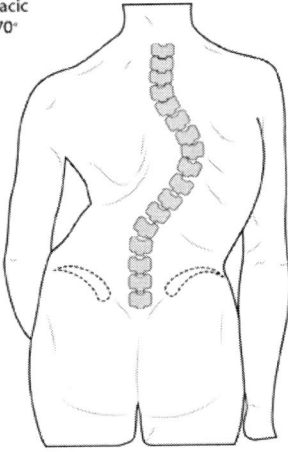

Right Thoracolumbar
Curver of 70°

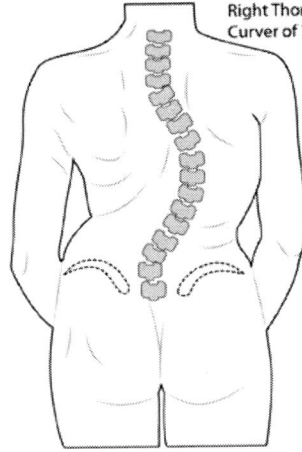

Left Lumbar
Curve of 70°
(Right Pelvic
Obliquity)

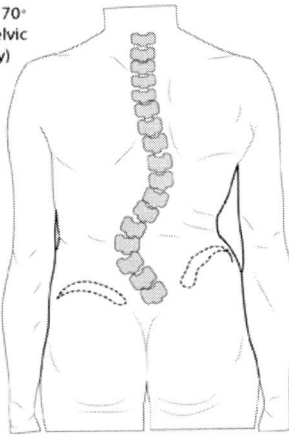

Double Major
Curve of 70°
(Right Thoracic
Left Lumbar)

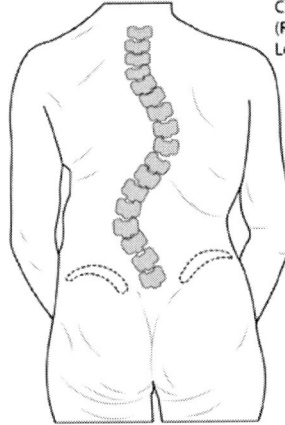

This series of drawings show how different the postural changes of scoliosis can appear.

One of the most common specific tests for detecting scoliosis is called the **Adam's Forward Bend Test** in which the individual bends from the waist as if touching their toes.

Adam's Forward Bend Test

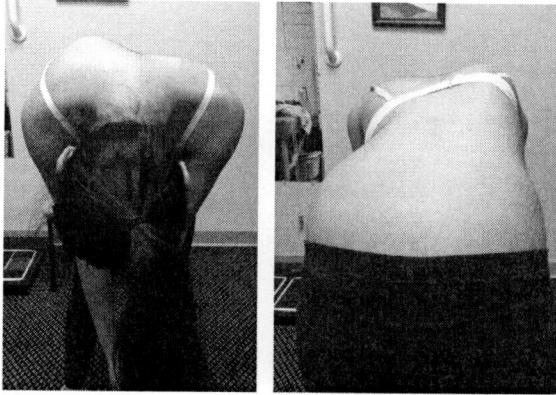

Although there are often few noticeable signs of scoliosis, one or more of the following indicators may show up:

Scoliosis Symptoms and Signs

- Shoulders may not be the same height (one higher than the other).

- Head is not centered directly above the pelvis.

- Rib cage is not symmetrical (ribs may be at different heights).

- One shoulder blade is higher and more prominent (it sticks out).

- One hip is more prominent (higher or sticking out).

- The individual may lean to one side.

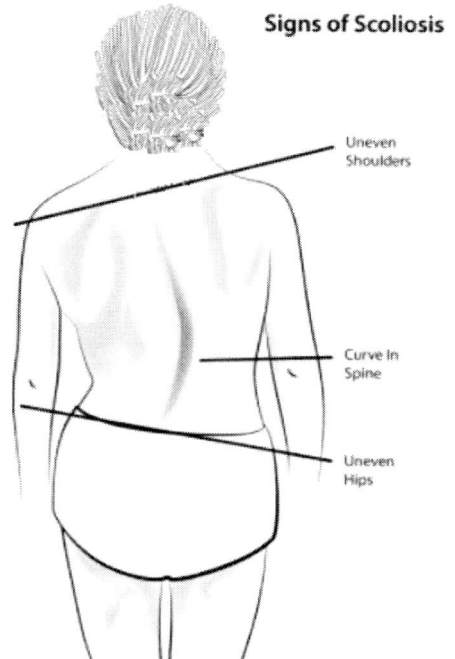

Signs of Scoliosis

Uneven Shoulders

Curve In Spine

Uneven Hips

- One leg may appear shorter than the other.

- The waist appears uneven.

- Clothes do not fit or hang properly.

- On the Adam's Forward Bend Test, one shoulder blade will protrude.

- The individual my look bent forward from a side view.

A tool called a "scoliometer" is used to measure the amount of trunk rotation which is a way to evaluate location and size of a curved spine.

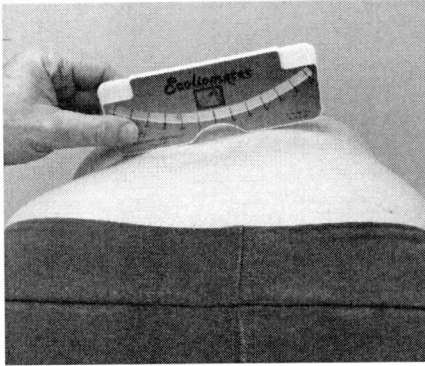

If you suspect you have scoliosis or have noticed any of the tell-tale signs, it is important to have an exam conducted by a scoliosis professional for proper diagnosis and possible treatment options.

> *In many spheres of human endeavor, from science to business to education to economic policy, good decisions depend on good measurement.*
>
> – Ben Bernanke

Chapter 4. How is a Scoliosis Measured?

Who was Cobb, and What is the Cobb Angle?

The **Cobb angle** was first described in 1948 by Dr. John R. Cobb, an American orthopedic surgeon, who used a unique technique to measure the angle of spinal curves. It is a measurement that evaluates scoliosis curves on a front-to-back x-ray of the spine. A variation of this procedure is also used to measure kyphosis and lordosis.[9]

How Does Someone Determine the Cobb Angle?

A curve is measured using the position of the **end/transitional vertebrae**. The **end vertebra** are the upper and lowermost vertebrae which are the least displaced from the midline and the most severely tilted.

A line is drawn along the **superior (top) endplate** of the **top end vertebra**, and a second line is drawn along the **inferior (bottom) end plate** of the **bottom end vertebra**. The angle formed by these two lines (or the lines drawn perpendicular to them) is the Cobb angle.

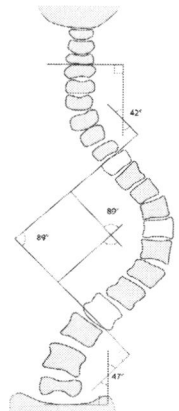

---

9 Cobb JR. "Outline for the study of scoliosis." *The American Academy of Orthopedic Surgeons Instructional Course Lectures.* Vol. 5. Ann Arbor, MI: Edwards; 1948.

For S-shaped scoliosis, where there are two curves, the bottom end vertebra of the upper curve will represent the top end vertebra of the lower curve.

What is the Significance of Cobb Angle?

The Cobb angle is a measure of the curvature of the spine in degrees, which helps the doctor to determine what type of treatment is necessary. It is an imperfect way to evaluate the scoliosis because it is measuring a three-dimensional distortion in only two dimensions. The scoliosis is a rotation or twist in the spine and can only be accurately measured by high-tech, high-radiation computerized tomography (CT). Scoliosis specialists have all agreed to rely on the Cobb method measured on an x-ray because it's low-tech, and the analysis requires a low amount of radiation.

Typically, a Cobb angle of 10 is regarded as a minimum curve size to define scoliosis. Does that mean someone with a nine-degree curvature does not have scoliosis? Bizarrely, even though this is an arbitrary designation, in the medical world the answer is "yes!"

Why Do Cobb Angles Appear to Vary?

Cobb angle is used worldwide to measure spinal abnormalities, particularly scoliosis. The Cobb angle measurement has become the gold standard of scoliosis evaluation and tracking and is endorsed by the Scoliosis Research Society.

The Adam's forward bend test is typically used as an important component of the scoliosis exam. If the test reveals signs of scoliosis, an x-ray is taken. If the x-ray indicates scoliosis, the Cobb angle is measured. However, because the Cobb angle reflects curvature only in a single plane, it fails to account for vertebral rotation, so it will not accurately demonstrate the severity of a three-dimensional spinal curvature.

Patients often ask, "Why does the Cobb angle calculation vary from doctor to doctor?" Like many medical tests, there is something called the "margin of error". **For Cobb measurement this means that the angle measured can**

vary from doctor to doctor by as much as 5 degrees. Another reason for Cobb angle variability is that patient placement at the time of the X-ray affects measurement.

That's why it is important to have the scoliosis evaluated beyond simply knowing a Cobb angle. Scoliosis is a three-dimensional distortion of the spine, and the care plan must reflect that reality of which Cobb angle is only a small part.

Look at the following images of a coat hanger. They reflect what happens when Cobb angles differ, depending on when, where and how they are determined. Looking at the hanger from different angles yields very different angle calculations – yet it's the same hanger.

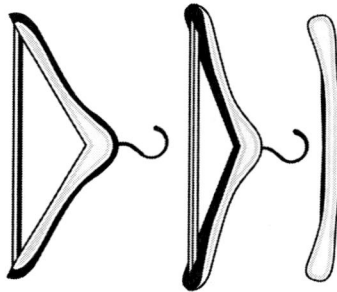

When a coat hanger is lying flat, the angle measures 60 degrees. If the coat hanger is rotated 90 degrees, the angle is zero. So, when the hanger is in between, the angle measures 30 degrees. This demonstrates how a patient's Cobb angle changes in degrees simply due to even slight rotation while the x-ray is being taken. Therefore, a curve correction from 60 degrees to 30 degrees, as the result of treatment, will represent significantly more than a 50 percent correction of the 3-D scoliosis.

Time of day also impacts the measurement of the Cobb angle. Marc Beauchamp and his research team published a study in a 1993 edition of *Spine*, showing that the measurement of a back curve could vary by up to 5 degrees – and even as much as 10-20 degrees in rare cases.[10]

10 Beauchamp, Marc et al. "Diurnal Variation of Cobb Angle Measurement in Adolescent Idiopathic Scoliosis." *Spine* 18.12 (1993): 1581-1583. 18 Apr. 2016

Chapter 5. Roundback (Kyphosis)

There are normal and abnormal spine curves. Although the spine should be straight when viewed from behind or from the front, it should exhibit normal curves when it is viewed from the side.

In a healthy back, the cervical (neck), thoracic (upper back) and lumbar (low back) segments of the spine are curved slightly. "**Kyphosis**" comes from the Greek word for "hump." Excessive curvature of the thoracic (middle) spine is known as "kyphosis" or the common terms **"roundback" or "hunchback."**

The individual bones or vertebrae that make up a healthy spine look like squares stacked to form a column. Kyphosis occurs when the

Good Posture   Thoracic Kyphosis / Hunchback

vertebrae in the upper back become more wedge shaped, curving the spine and causing the spinal column to lose some — or all — of its normal curvature. This causes a bowing of the back, seen as a slouching posture.

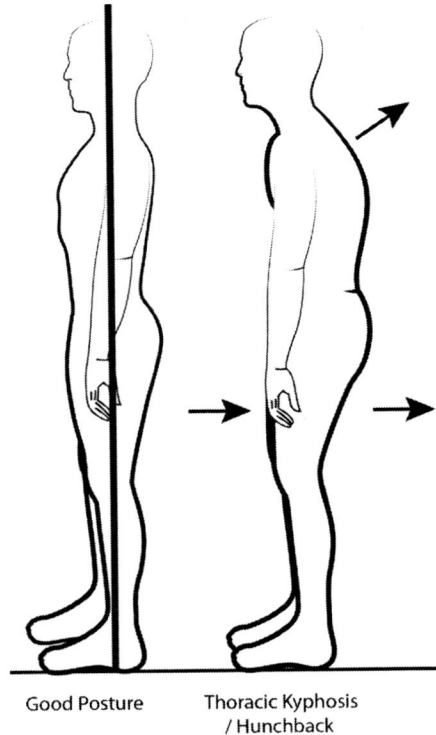

While most cases of kyphosis are mild and can b easily improved with postural exercises, serious cases can be debilitating. High degrees of kyphosis can cause a distressing hunched-forward cosmetic deformity, as well as severe pain and discomfort, breathing and digestion difficulties, cardiovascular irregularities, reduced height, difficulty standing upright, neurological compromise, and even significantly shortened life spans in the more severe cases.

Kyphosis can begin at any age and affects both men and women. Most commonly found in the upper back, it is possible to develop kyphosis in the neck or low back.

Types of Kyphosis

Postural kyphosis is the most common type and can be found in children and adults. It is commonly attributed to slouching and may be reversible by correcting muscular imbalances. Kyphosis development in children can be improved with postural exercises along with the posture awareness associated with regular sports like dance, yoga, or martial arts. In adult patients, it is referred to as **"hyperkyphosis,"** **or "dowager's hump."** It indicates a Cobb angle greater than 40 degrees and is most common in older women. If the curve angle exceeds 70—75 degrees, many surgeons will recommend a complex surgery to reduce the kyphosis. Hyperkyphosis can develop due to aging alone, but about one-third of the most severe hyperkyphosis cases occur after osteoporosis weakens spinal bones to the point that they crack and compress.

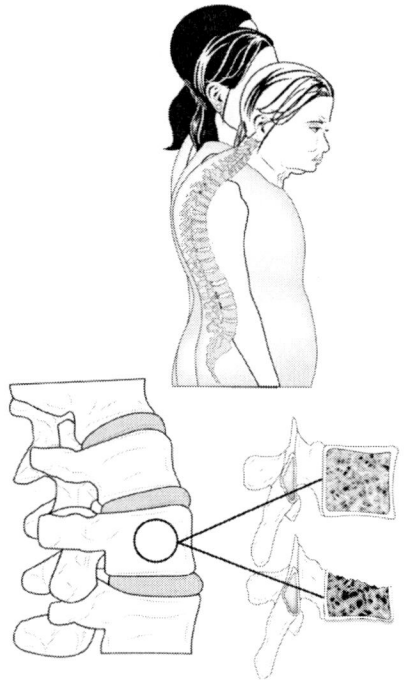

Scheuermann's kyphosis is a disease that can lead to significant deformity. It can cause varying degrees of pain and can affect different regions of the spine. It is most commonly found in the mid-thoracic region.

More commonly referred to as "**Scheuermann's disease,**" it is found mostly in teenagers. Boys are affected more often than girls. A patient with Scheuermann's kyphosis cannot consciously correct posture because the curved part of the spine is very rigid. The patient may feel pain in this area, which can be aggravated by physical activity and long periods of standing or sitting. Whereas the vertebrae and disks appear normal in postural kyphosis, these structures in Scheuermann's kyphosis are irregular, often herniated, and wedge-shaped on at least three adjacent levels. Mild scoliosis commonly accompanies Scheuermann's kyphosis.

Fatigue is a very common symptom, most likely because of the intense muscle work required to stand or sit properly. The condition appears to be hereditary. Most of the patients who undergo surgery to correct their kyphosis have Scheuermann's disease. In patients with between 45 and 70 degrees of curvature, where skeletal growth is still occurring, bracing and a specific exercise program have been shown to be a successful treatment plan. In older patients, kyphosis-specific exercises along with end-of-day bracing has been shown to relieve pain, stabilize the kyphosis, but not to correct the condition.

Congenital kyphosis occurs in rare cases in which an infant's spinal column does not develop correctly in the womb. Vertebrae may be malformed or fused together and can cause progressive kyphosis as the child develops. Surgical treatment may be necessary at a very early stage, and consistent follow-up will be an important part of maintaining a normal curve. However, the decision to carry out the procedure can be very difficult, due to potential risks to the child (similar to the risks associated with any spine surgery, see Chapter 23). A congenital kyphosis also can appear suddenly in teenage years — more commonly in children with cerebral palsy and other neurological disorders.

Nutritional kyphosis can result from deficiencies in the diet, especially during childhood. A vitamin D or calcium deficiency, for example, can cause rickets, a softening of the bones that results in curving of the spine and limbs under the child's body weight. In adults, this is referred to as osteomalacia.[11]

Gibbus deformity is a form of structural kyphosis, where one or more adjacent vertebrae become wedged. Gibbus deformity can result from advanced skeletal tuberculosis or severe osteoporosis and is caused by collapsed vertebral bodies. This can lead to spinal cord compression causing paraplegia, an impairment in motor or sensory function of the lower extremities.

The most common cause of kyphosis in the elderly is due to vertebral fracture caused by **osteoporosis.** *Osteoporosis can be found in both males and females but is more common in women. Osteoporosis weakens the bones, making them susceptible to fracture. A fracture of the bones of the spine changes the shape of the spinal bones from that of a cube to a wedge with the front of the wedge toward the front of the body. This causes the body to tip forward into a stooped posture.*

Post-traumatic kyphosis occurs from untreated or ineffectively treated vertebral fractures or severe injuries to the ligaments of the spine.

Camptocormia (also known as bent spine syndrome) is an abnormal bent-over position of the trunk that is very obvious when the person is standing and especially obvious when walking, but completely disappears when they lie down. Mostly seen in elderly patients, the condition is often related to a wasting of the back muscles, but the underlying cause is not known. There are many named diseases that can cause this type of muscular weakness and they must be ruled out by appropriate testing, most commonly MRI scanning. There is no drug therapy for idiopathic camptocormia and therapy along with exercise must be encouraged.

Neuromuscular kyphosis is a deformity that begins in childhood when there is cerebral palsy, muscular dystrophy or spina bifida.

---

11 Sahay, M. "Rickets–Vitamin D Deficiency and Dependency - NCBI." 2012. 26 Apr. 2016 http://www.ncbi.nlm.nih.gov/pmc/articles/PMC3313732/

Degenerative kyphosis is due to excessive wear and tear of the bones of the spine over a long period of time. Commonly this is a result of osteoarthritis with degenerative changes to the spinal discs.

Kyphosis Diagnosis

For kyphosis diagnosis, a physical examination is required. A health-care provider will check height and may ask the patient to bend forward from the waist while the provider views the spine from the side. The rounding of the upper back may become more obvious in this position. Reflexes and muscle strength will be checked, and depending on symptoms, x-rays may be ordered. These tests will help determine the degree of curvature, if there are any deformities of the vertebrae, and identify the type of kyphosis if it is present. If there is numbness or muscle weakness, the doctor may recommend tests to determine how well nerve impulses are traveling between the spinal cord and extremities. If the kyphosis is severe, the doctor may check for breathing interference using **"spirometry,"** a lung function test.

Kyphosis Treatment in Adults

Kyphosis treatment depends upon age, cause and effects. Kyphosis also may cause back pain and stiffness in some people. Mild cases of kyphosis may produce no noticeable signs or symptoms. Stretching exercises can improve spinal flexibility in mild cases of **postural kyphosis**. Exercises that strengthen the abdominal muscles may help improve posture, too.

The discomfort and strain of structural kyphosis can be helped by performing specific strengthening exercises, active self-correction, targeted stretching, neuromuscular re-education, and, in more severe cases, a kyphosis brace that is usually prescribed to be worn six or more hours each day. The program of care in most cases can improve spine mobility significantly and reduce postural distortions. The program can reduce or eliminate pain as well as slow or stop kyphosis progression. In selected adult patients, there can be a modest reduction in the overall size of the kyphosis.

If the kyphosis curve is severe, particularly if the spinal bones are protruding or herniated discs are pinching the spinal cord or nerve roots, surgery may be prescribed. Spinal fusion surgery connects two or more of the affected vertebrae permanently. Surgeons insert bits of bone between the vertebrae and then fasten the vertebrae together with metal wires, plates and screws. The complication rate for spinal surgery is relatively high, and problems may include bleeding, infection, pain, nerve damage, arthritis, and disk degeneration. Follow up surgeries may be needed.

Chapter 6. Swayback (Lordosis)

Remember that a normal spine, when viewed from behind, appears straight. From the side, the spine normally curves at the neck, the torso, and the lower-back area. This positions the head over the pelvis naturally. These curves also work as shock absorbers that distribute the stress that occurs during walking, lifting, and bending.

Normal spinal contours are essential for the correct biomechanics of the spine. Nature designed the spine as a marvelous machine combining the strength of a column with the flexibility of a spring.

Lordosis is the inward curvature of a portion of the lumbar (low back) and cervical (neck) spine. In a spine affected by **hyperlordosis, or excessive lordosis**, the vertebrae of the low back form an excessively curved or swayback appearance.

A major aspect of this spinal distortion is excessive **anterior pelvic tilt**, in which the pelvis tips forward as it is resting on top of the femurs (thigh bones). When lying face up on a hard surface, a large degree of lordosis will appear as a space under the lower back.

Excessive lordosis may increase at puberty, although it is sometimes not evident until the early or mid-20s. Excessive lordosis, or **hyperlordosis**, is commonly referred to as **"hollow back," "sway back"** or **"saddle back,"** a term that originates from the similar condition that arises in some horses.

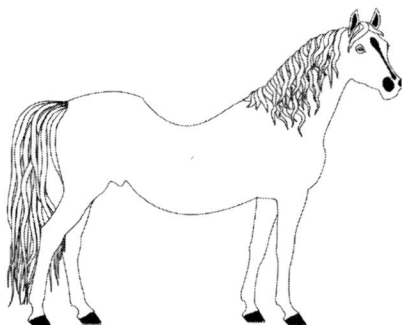

A reduction in the normal lower-back curve is called "**hypo**lordosis."

This loss of normal lordosis will cause a stretching of the disc towards the back, compressing it towards the front and potentially causing a narrowing of the opening for the nerves, possibly pinching them.

In the neck, a loss of lordosis creates joint instability and pitches the head forward. The weight of the head (10-12 lbs) being placed forward of its normal position, combined with joint instability, causes muscle tension and strain on the neck, upper back, and shoulders. Headache under that base of the skull is a common effect of forward head position.

Symptoms of Swayback & Flatback

Hyper (too much) or **Hypo** (too little) lordosis can lead to moderate-to-severe lower back pain and cause pain that affects the ability to move. If the curve is flexible (reverses itself when the person bends forward), there is

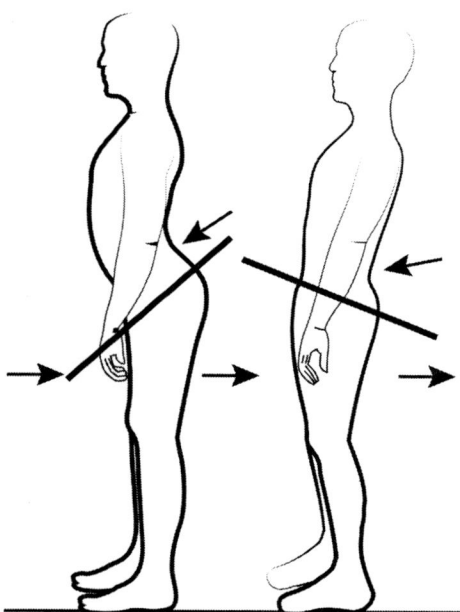

Lumbar Lordosis
/ Anterior Pelvic Tilt
/ Swayback

Flat back
/ Posterior Pelvic Tilt

little need for concern. If the curve does not change when the person bends forward, the lordosis is fixed or locked, and treatment is needed.

Causes of Lordosis

Hyperlordosis affects people of all ages. It is common in dancers and gymnasts, and certain conditions can contribute to lordosis, including, kyphosis, pregnancy, osteoporosis and excessive belly fat. A heavy belly may pull the pelvis to the front, tilting the spine too much. Imbalances in muscle strength and muscle length are also a cause. Tight lower back muscles, weak hamstrings and overly tight hip flexors may aggravate the condition. Rickets or osteomalacia, a vitamin D deficiency, also can cause lumbar **hyper**lordosis.

Hypolordosis is commonly found in adults with adolescent idiopathic scoliosis (ASA) and almost universally in adult de novo scoliosis patients.

Lordosis Diagnosis

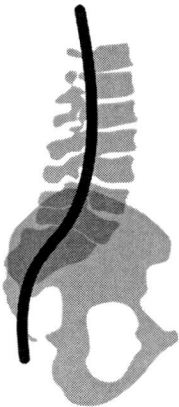

Lordotic Lumbar Spine

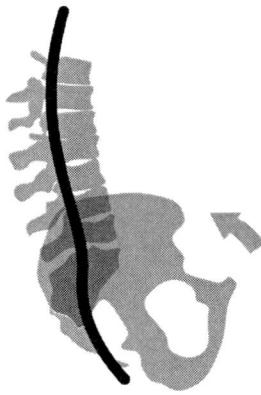

Kyphotic Lumbar Spine

To diagnose lordosis, the patient's medical history and a physical exam are necessary, especially if excessive or diminished curve becomes noticeable or seems to be getting worse. The patient will be asked to bend forward and to the side to see whether the curve is flexible or fixed, how much range of motion the patient has, and if the spine is aligned properly. The doctor will feel the spine to check for abnormalities like poor joint alignment, muscle spasm, fixation of the joints, heat indicating inflammation of the joints, and painful regions.

A neurological assessment (including Electromyography) may be necessary if the person is having pain, tingling, numbness, muscle spasms, or weakness, sensations in his or her arms or legs, or changes in bowel or bladder control. X-rays (or MRI) may be taken of the whole back or just the lower back.

Treatment for Lordosis

Lordosis treatment involves similar principles of home exercise as for cases of adult scoliosis, but with a different emphasis. Isometrics are used to build strength. Targeted stretching is employed to improve flexibility and increase range of motion. **Lumbar lordosis treatment** consists of strengthening muscles on the back of the thighs and stretching the group of muscles on the front of the thighs. The muscles on the front and on the back of the thighs can rotate the pelvis forward or backward while in a standing position because they can discharge the force on the ground through the legs and feet.

An active self-correction program is developed to train the patient to assume a more normal posture during their daily activities of sitting and standing. This is a powerful technique to stabilize the spine in cases of hyper and hypo lordosis.

Neuromuscular re-education techniques are used to retrain the brain to hold the corrected posture. This is done by placing weights on the body while standing on an unstable surface like a foam mat or a balance disc.

The very common finding of hypolordosis in adult degenerative scoliosis (de novo scoliosis) is thought to be due to the body's reaction to instability in the spine caused by lack of the normal ligament strength. The body tightens the adjacent muscles in a protective reaction to the instability. Unfortunately, the loss of lordosis places additional strain on the spine and a vicious cycle of progressively worsening scoliosis and degeneration often results. Part of scoliosis care must be to protect and augment the normal spinal contours.

One of the biggest criticisms of scoliosis surgery (both for children and adults) is that certain techniques can cause a loss of normal curves in both the neck and back, which then weakens the spine.

Hypolordosis can be improved non-surgically through the four-part rehabilitation exercise program. If done correctly, symptoms can be reduced in
three to six months. If excess belly fat is contributing to the hyperlordosis,
weight loss may be required to decrease the curve. Only the most severe
cases of lordosis require surgery, which may involve spinal instrumentation, artificial disc replacement, and kyphoplasty – the surgical filling of an
injured or collapsed vertebra.

Like with scoliosis, early detection is key to treating lordosis.

> *Time and health are two precious assets that we don't recognize and appreciate until they have been depleted.*
>
> **– Denis Waitley**

Chapter 7. The 2 Types of Adult Scoliosis

Adolescent Scoliosis in an Adult (ASA)

Once skeletal maturity is reached, a patient with adolescent idiopathic scoliosis is now labeled as having **adolescent scoliosis in an adult (ASA).**[12] There is typically a slow increase (about 0.3-1 degree per year) in the curvature[13] that began during teen years in an otherwise healthy individual which is progressive during adult life.[14]

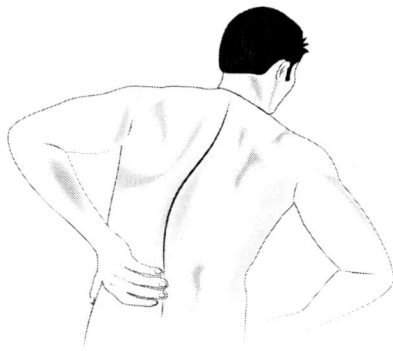

These curves can occur in the thoracic (upper) and lumbar (lower) spine and have the same basic appearance as those seen with adolescent scoliosis. Physical symptoms can include: shoulder asymmetry, a rib hump, or a prominence of the lower back on the side of the curvature.

---

12 "Adults with Idiopathic Scoliosis Improve Disability ... – Springer." 2016. 11 Apr. 2016 http://link.springer.com/content/pdf/10.1007 percent2Fs00586-016-4528-y.pdf

13 Negrini, A. "Scoliosis-Specific Exercises Can Reduce the Progression of ..." 2015. 26 Apr. 2016 http://www.ncbi.nlm.nih.gov/pmc/articles/PMC4537533/

14 Choudhry MN, Ahmad Z, Verma R (2016) Adolescent idiopathic scoliosis. *Open Orthop J* 10:143–154 https://www.ncbi.nlm.nih.gov/pmc/articles/PMC4897334/

Adult-Onset, Degenerative De Novo Scoliosis (DDS)

Not to be confused with Adult Idiopathic Scoliosis, **Adult Scoliosis** or **Adult-Onset Scoliosis** (also known as De Novo Scoliosis) is a degenerative scoliosis, or a side-to-side curvature of the spine associated with by breakdown of the small joints of the spine.

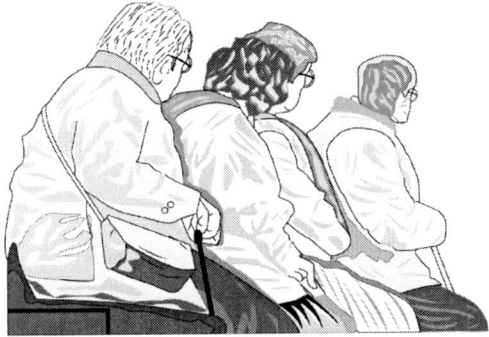

The prevalence of scoliosis among adolescents is 4 percent. Surprisingly, in adults in general, scoliosis prevalence is over 20 percent. It increases to 40 percent in adults over age 60 and to 68 percent in adults over age 70. Two thirds of the elderly population has scoliosis, AND pain associated with scoliosis is common in older patients. Degenerative scoliosis is found only in older adults, most frequently in people over age 50. Adult-onset scoliosis affects more of the spine, including the neck. Typically, a C curve scoliosis forms in the lumbar spine. It can occur due to degeneration in the spine, also known as **Spondylosis.**

Weakening of the normal ligaments and other soft tissues of the spine combined with abnormal bone spurs can lead to an abnormal curvature of the spine. The spine can also be affected by osteoporosis, vertebral compression fractures, and disc degeneration. The pain of the underlying cause of this type of scoliosis causes people to lean to one side, to reduce pressure on the area or as an effect of the body weight being shifted, causing spinal deformity.

Degenerative scoliosis is the most common form of scoliosis in adults. The prevalence of adult scoliosis (de novo) is increasing in North America due to the demographic shifts of an aging population, associated with an increased life expectancy.

What Causes Degenerative Scoliosis?

Degenerative scoliosis is caused by a gradual deterioration of the **facet joints** (small stabilizing joints of the spine located between and behind adjacent vertebrae). This is the same process of gradual wear and tear that causes osteoarthritis of the spine. However, in degenerative scoliosis, the pressure of these deteriorating facet joints causes a straight spine (when viewed from behind) to become crooked.

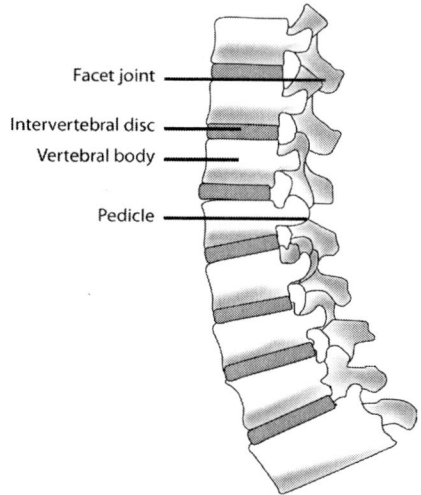

Facet joint

Intervertebral disc
Vertebral body

Pedicle

What are the Symptoms of Adult-Onset Scoliosis?

As we get older, cartilage in the joints can naturally erode. In the spine, this cartilage in the facet joints contributes to the spine's flexibility. When the facet joints deteriorate, it can become painful for the spine to flex and bend as usual. Without the protective cartilage, the joints become irritated and inflamed causing pain. Pain is present in some patients, but not all. Patients may experience stiffness and pain in the mid to lower back and/or pain, numbness, and weakness in the legs and feet. Some patients will not have much pain, and are more concerned about the postural shift and the way it affects how they look.

Back pain from degenerative scoliosis comes on gradually and worsens over time. The pain is typically worse in the morning, improves slightly once the patient has become more active, and then worsens at the end of the day. Typically, sitting provides more comfort than standing or walking because the facet joints receive less pressure in this position. As the facet joints get irritated and inflamed, they aggravate lumbar stenosis, a narrowing of the spinal canal in the lower back. Nerve root inflammation can cause further constriction. These nerve roots affect the legs and therefore leg pain in one or both legs can be felt when standing or walking.

Let's Review What Signs to Look for When Adult Scoliosis is Suspected:

- Shoulders may not be the same height.

- Head is not centered above the pelvis.

- Ribs may be at different heights.

- A shoulder blade may stick out.

- The individual may lean to one side.

- One leg may appear shorter.

- The waist appears uneven.

- Clothes do not fit/hang properly.

- Flattening of the lower back or "hypolordosis."

ASA has a very similar presentation to AIS, but de novo scoliosis will present more typically with only lumbar (lower back) scoliosis. It can be very difficult to distinguish de novo from ASA. Often the only absolute determiner of ASA vs de novo is that the patient describes having scoliosis as a teen!

If the scoliosis is in the upper back, a physical examination will reveal a more prominent shoulder blade when the patient bends forward. You may recall that this is called an "Adam's forward bend test." Often the spine curves to the right in the upper back and to the left in the lower back, causing the right shoulder to be higher than the left. If the scoliosis is in the lower back, one hip may be more prominent than the other. X-rays taken while the patient is standing will confirm the extent and type of scoliosis.

It can be challenging to determine what initially caused the curvature, once it has significantly progressed. However, if there is asymmetric (uneven) degeneration, this leads to greater asymmetric load (uneven weight distribution) and progression of the degeneration and deformity, in the form of scoliosis and/or kyphosis. In postmenopausal women, progression can increase due to osteoporosis. Degradation of the facet joints, joint capsules, discs and ligaments leads to mono- or multi-segmental instability (greater than normal range of motion (or "hypermobility") between vertebral segments) leading to spinal stenosis.

How is Adolescent Scoliosis in an Adult Treated?

While an adult with scoliosis will greatly benefit from adult scoliosis exercises to stop progression, pain is a much more common reason to seek treatment. Pain control must be the top priority of all conservative scoliosis care programs. Commonly, patients present for care who were diagnosed with idiopathic scoliosis earlier in life, but were not prescribed treatment because their curves were not deemed severe enough to warrant the standard medical approach of bracing or surgery. These patients later find that by adulthood their curves have either progressed so that they now are causing significant postural distortions and/or now cause pain. Other patients may have been braced with older brace designs during adolescence only to have their "corrected" curves deteriorate and or continue to progress as adults.

Adult scoliosis patients differ from adolescent patients because the curves tend to cause back pain – often the main complaint. The curves also tend to be rigid, more severe and progressive, making treatment more challenging. Advanced stages of disc degeneration are also associated with adult scoliosis and may be the primary reason for back pain in many patients. Pinched nerves from herniated discs and arthritic changes may also be a challenge. In late middle age and after, it is common for patients to develop osteopenia (low bone density) or osteoporosis – factors which affect treatment. Because normal degenerative changes of the spine may be accelerated by a spinal curvature, the older patient may be at higher risk for skeletal pain or extremity pain from nerve compression.

It is important to have a specialist in adult scoliosis monitor the curve because these curves can worsen due to the disc degeneration and increasing postural distortions. This also may cause patients to lean progressively forward. This forward shift in posture is the greatest predictor of pain and disability in adults with scoliosis.

> *Pain and disability more commonly determine treatment decisions for older patients with scoliosis, while the deformity typically guides treatment planning for younger scoliosis patients.*

How is De Novo Scoliosis Treated?

Since degenerative scoliosis is caused by the deterioration of the joints in the spine due to aging, the curve that results from this typically progresses 1, 2 or even 3 degrees per year. It is often the inflammation of the degenerated spinal joints, and the associated disc damage, and postural strain that causes a majority of the spinal pain. Treatment is focused on both managing pain as well as stopping curve progression.

With age, the correction that can be achieved will be limited by any severe degenerative (arthritic) changes in the spine. The first priority is always to eliminate pain, then stop curve progression, improve posture and cosmetic appearance, and ultimately — to a more limited extent than in an adolescent —reduce the size of the curve.

Elderly individuals with degenerative scoliosis may need to avoid or modify activities that aggravate symptoms and cause pain.

Your specialized scoliosis exercise doctor will recommend adult scoliosis treatment, specifically designed for older adults with scoliosis. This will include adult scoliosis exercises that will improve scoliosis by stabilizing the spine and correcting imbalances that are causing the spine to curve. Along with active self-correction maneuvers and carefully targeted stretching techniques individually tailored to each patient's unique needs, elderly scoliosis patients can also benefit from gentle chiropractic treatments.

Patients with severe scoliosis (curves greater than 60 degrees) may rarely be candidates for surgery, but of course the risks associated with surgery increase with the age of the patient. Surgery is indicated when the patient describes unbearable pain through which they cannot perform their normal daily functions, loss of control of the bowels or bladder, or withering of an arm or leg. These are surgical emergencies and conservative exercise-based care is no longer appropriate.

If you are elderly, do not give up! In most cases, pain can still be greatly reduced or even eliminated and prevented from recurring, AND curves can be stabilized.

Traditionally adult scoliosis has been treated with a watch-and-wait philosophy. Patients have been given pain medications, as needed, and surgery has been viewed as the option of last resort only if the patient had unmanageable, severe pain, loss of control of the bowel or bladder, or withering of the arms and or legs.

That Was Then. This Is Now!

Now, there is a more proactive approach than the previous wait-and-see method of pain medications. Keep in mind that it is important to treat scoliosis curves **BEFORE** they progress to surgical levels, rather than **AFTER**. Not only are there more treatment options that address scoliosis early on, but there are also non-invasive treatments that do not employ the use of surgery.

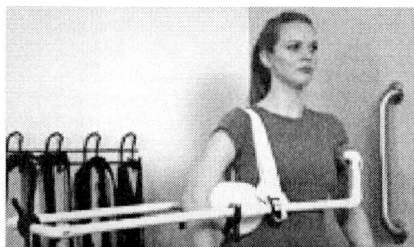

Modern home-care programs use custom-designed scoliosis exercises consisting of spinal resistance training in conjunction with the principles of specific brain-retraining maneuvers to restore the spine's alignment. Each unique adult scoliosis patient is treated with a **customized program** of neuromuscular re-education that includes scoliosis specific exercises, targeted stretching, and active self-correction methods. Early intervention is essential to reduce the curve and avoid the difficulties inherent in large-curve treatment.

In the recent past, only infantile, juvenile, or adolescent idiopathic scoliosis was treated with scoliosis bracing. Now, adult scoliosis bracing is being used as an effective treatment for controlling pain, improving posture, and limiting or halting progression. Bracing is not recommended for all adult scoliosis cases. Roughly 20 percent to 30 percent of adult cases may benefit from adult scoliosis bracing.

While ANY scoliosis treatment programs (including exercise-based, bracing or surgery) may not eliminate scoliosis completely, they will reduce and stabilize the curve. It is fine for an adult to have a mild scoliosis and continue to use a custom-designed home-exercise program as they continue to age. This gives them the power to control the condition themselves. What is important is that they have a customized program of home care they can use to stabilize the spine, reduce or eliminate the pain, and slow or stop progression. Now they are in control of their scoliosis AND are providing themselves with the best chance to ultimately avoid surgery!

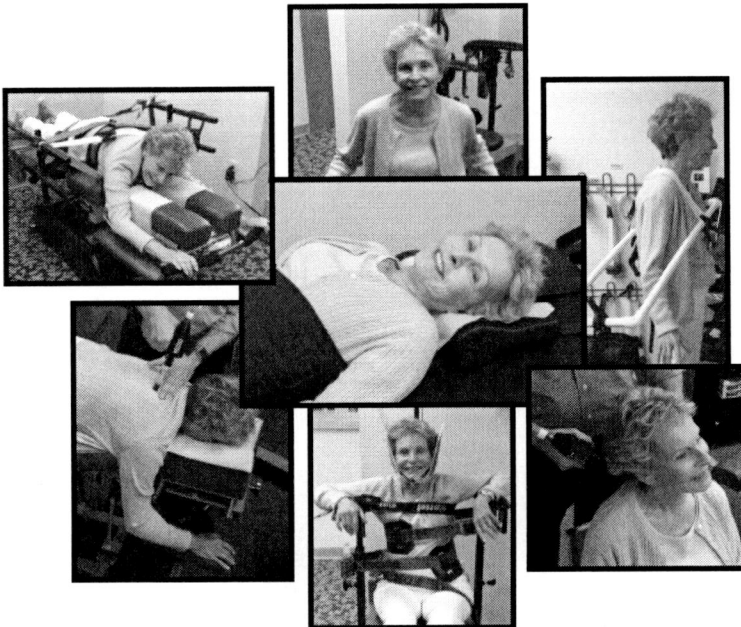

First, use a custom-designed, exercise-based home program. Then consider corrective bracing. Only as a last resort should the patient submit to a surgical correction.

This just makes sense!

Chapter 8. 'Mild Scoliosis' and it's Possible Progression in Adults

Mild scoliosis is a 10- to 20-degree Cobb Angle. Research tells us that mild scoliosis has a 22 percent chance of progressing. This is a significant risk. Once the scoliosis passes the 20-degree mark, risk of progression more than triples to 68 percent!

Symptoms of Mild Scoliosis

- Scoliosis curve is less than 20 degrees.

- May have tilted head, uneven shoulders or hips.

- Head may appear more forward than shoulders when viewed from the side (forward head posture).

- Clothing may hang unevenly.

- May have uneven leg lengths.

- May not be observable from posture, even by physicians.

- May or may not be accompanied by pain.

Mild Scoliosis Treatment

- Easier to treat when the curve is small

- Overwhelmingly the research[15] shows that mild curves respond well to scoliosis-specific, exercise-based correction programs without the need for bracing in most cases. To achieve this impressive result, it is vital to remove the underlying causes of the scoliosis before the 30-degree mark occurs. The appropriate custom-designed program of targeted stretching, neurological re-education, active self-correction techniques, along with isometric and isotonic exercises, will maintain the upper hand against the forces attempting to drive curve progression.

> *"All LARGE Scoliosis Curves Have One Thing in Common.*
> *They Started as small Curves."*

Why Early Scoliosis Intervention is Crucial

It can be nearly impossible to tell just by looking at a person whether they have scoliosis. This is often the case for mild scoliosis patients. Adults often contact my office with a similar tale of being unaware of their scoliosis during childhood or even the majority of their late years and then finding out they have a large curve. This curve was obviously many years in development but was never diagnosed.

While scoliosis appears to be a side-to-side curve in the spine, it's actually a twisting of the spine around its axis causing the rib cage to rotate as well. This twisting of the spine can gradually cause a severe torque that makes the existing spinal curve twist and bend even more. The effect becomes visible when the torso is pushed to one side causing a "rib hump." These postural changes can start to occur before the Cobb angle measurement would indicate a significant problem. When treatment is initiated while the curve is still small there is a far greater chance of a successful outcome.

---

15 Negrini, S., et al. "2016 SOSORT guidelines: orthopaedic and rehabilitation treatment of idiopathic scoliosis during growth." Scoliosis and Spinal Disorders. 2018;13:3. https://scoliosisjournal.biomedcentral.com/articles/10.1186/s13013-017-0145-8

What does the Research Say About Progression in Adults?

- Danielson and Nachemson (*Spine* 2003) found that 36 percent of adolescents with scoliosis had progressed by more than 10 degrees after 22 years.

- Chopin et al. found the average curve progression by type the type of adult scoliosis:

  - lumbar curves 1.8 degrees /yr

  - thoracolumbar curves 1.4 degrees /yr

  - thoracic curves 1.2 degrees /yr

  - double curves thoracic 0.8 degrees /yr

- Degenerative de novo scoliosis DDS Avg 3 degrees /yr

Chin, Furey, and Bohlman[16] listed the risk factors that lead to curve size progression in adults with a mild scoliosis:

1. Reduction of the normal lower back curve.

2. Significant side slippage (lateral listhesis) of more than 5mm.

3. Sex (females more likely than males).

4. Age (increasing age leads to higher risk).

5. Curve shape (large lower back curves are a higher risk).

6. Imbalance of the pelvic bones.

They concluded that small curves can progress and therefore should be treated on an individualized context.

---

16 Chin KR, Furey C, Bohlman HH. "Risk of progression in de novo low-magnitude degenerative lumbar curves: natural history and literature review." *American Journal of Orthopedics.* (Belle Mead NJ). 2009 Aug;38(8):404-9. https://www.ncbi.nlm.nih.gov/pubmed/19809605

Let's now look at a very well-respected study[17] on what happens to untreated adult scoliosis as the patient ages.

- 51 scoliosis patients – 48 females, 3 males

- Mean age at first X-ray 37 years (17-60)

- All but 8 of the patients reported low back pain

- 22 reported nerve root pain

- 4 were pain-free

- Overall, there were 51 thoracolumbar and lumbar curves, including 30 single major curves

The chart below summarizes the study's conclusions. The two types of adult scoliosis described in this study:

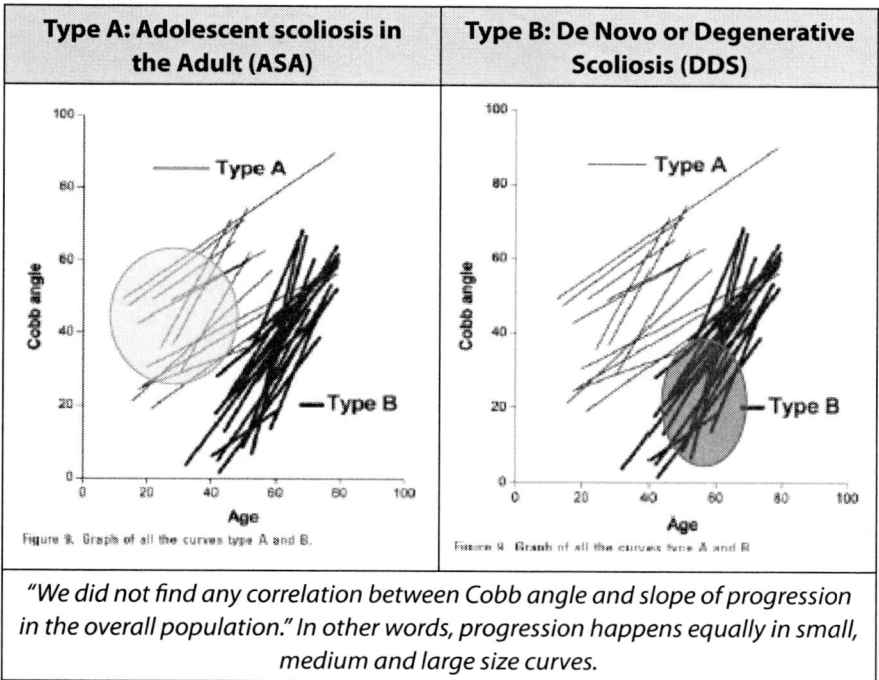

Type A: Adolescent scoliosis in the Adult (ASA)	Type B: De Novo or Degenerative Scoliosis (DDS)
Figure 3. Graph of all the curves type A and B.	Figure 3. Graph of all the curves type A and B.
"We did not find any correlation between Cobb angle and slope of progression in the overall population." In other words, progression happens equally in small, medium and large size curves.	

17 Marty-Poumarat et.al. (Spine 2007) Natural History of Progressive Adult Scoliosis.

This key finding shows that even smaller curves are progressive in adulthood.

Marty-Poumarat also looked at the role menopause plays:

- Among those with ASA, 8 women with a long-time period of gradual progression showed no change in the rate of progression at menopause.

- Patients with DDS were all women with single lumbar or thoracolumbar curves.

- In those with DDS, 11 out of 20 saw more rapid progression at the time of menopause.

Summary of the Study Findings:

- The progression of adult scoliosis is a predictable and steadily increase in curve size.

- Twisting of the bones with pinching of the nerves is an initial factor of progression for DDS but is the consequence of progression for ASA.

- Menopause is a period of deterioration for DDS but not for ASA.

> *No one can avoid aging, but aging productively is something else.*
>
> – **Katharine Graham**

Chapter 9. Lateral Listhesis

As the adult scoliosis spine ages, the spine and its supporting ligaments weaken and degenerate, and the vertebrae begin to twist and shift to the side. This is called a **Lateral Listhesis.** This slippage raises concerns about the possibility of postural collapse.

De novo scoliosis usually presents with combined loss of lordosis (normal curvature of the low back), AND often a shifting of the vertebrae due to breakdown of the spinal joints. Although the underlying cause is not fully understood, degenerative scoliosis is associated with degenerative disc disease, failure of the small joints at the back of the spine, and a thickening of the major ligaments that are attempting to support the weakened spinal bones.

This type of curvature with degeneration can lead to nerve pain radiating down the legs, along with strong lower back pain, and can eventually lead to a dangerous condition called postural collapse. Early treatment with a scoliosis specific exercise program and possibly adult scoliosis bracing is the best approach. Surgery can be considered in more severe cases, but the benefits and risks to the patient must be carefully considered before that choice is made.

Let's look more closely at the underlying structures and changes that lead to this problem.

Spinal Joint Instability

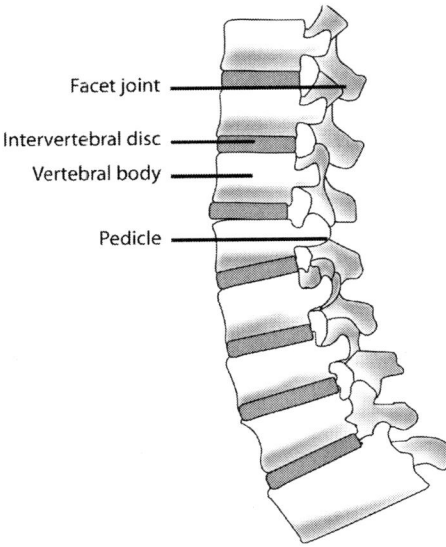

Facet joint

Intervertebral disc

Vertebral body

Pedicle

Spinal joint instability is abnormal excessive movement (or "hypermobility") between two vertebrae (bones of the spine).

Between the vertebrae are intervertebral discs and stabilizing ligaments. The discs and ligaments hold the vertebrae together, forming stable strong joints that allow slight movement between the vertebrae with the disc also functioning as a shock absorber. As all people get older, they will experience decreased back support due to normal changes to the aging spine. Greater force is placed on the discs, which then accelerates degenerative disc disease. When a disc narrows from degeneration in the presence of scoliosis, the bones above and below the disc move or slip on each other causing the vertebrae to shift either forward, backward or (most importantly for adult scoliosis patients) the vertebrae can slip to the side severely weakening the spine. This movement indicates "segmental spinal instability."

Disc degeneration is associated with a loss of ligamentous strength. This weakness causes increased movement between the vertebrae. Increased movement along with a decrease in the disc height allows the spinal joints to move out of alignment.

The breakdown of structural spinal elements like discs, supportive ligaments, facet joints, and joint lubricating capsules responsible for stability, leads to multi-directional instability effecting two or more spinal bones. Depending on the direction and location, this misalignment can be diagnosed as **spondylolisthesis** (forward slippage)**, lateral listhesis** (side slippage) or **retrolisthesis** (backward slippage).

Spondylolisthesis (forward slippage)

Also called an **anterolisthesis,** translational or rotary **olisthesis,** it is an anterior (forward) slip of lumbar vertebrae (most often the fifth lumbar vertebra) and sometimes cervical vertebrae. About 5 percent to 7 percent of all people (with or without scoliosis) are affected by spondylolisthesis. The two main causes are from either a stress fracture in the vertebrae called **spondylolysis,** or by degeneration of the facet joints. It is often caused or aggravated by certain sports (repeated trauma) or it can be caused by an isolated incident (an accident or fall). When spondylolisthesis occurs with scoliosis, it is sometimes referred to as **"olisthesis".**

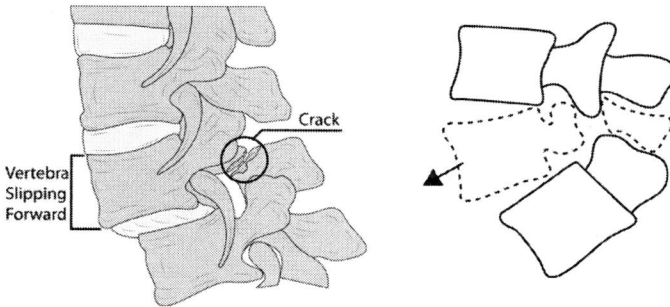

Retrolisthesis

Posterior (backward) slip of lumbar vertebrae brought on by the same mechanisms as spondylolisthesis (mentioned above).

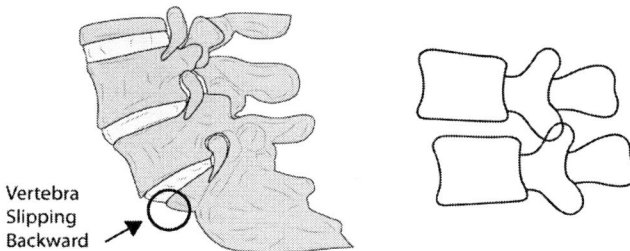

Lateral listhesis

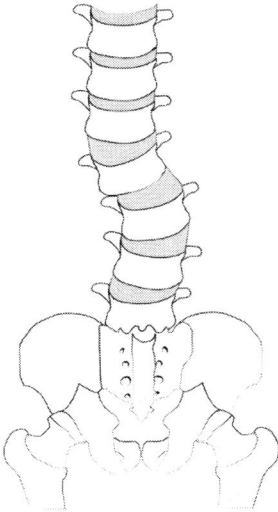

Also known as **rotatory subluxation**, this is when one vertebra slides off another vertebra in both the coronal (front to back) and axial planes (top to bottom). Due to the effects of gravity, quite commonly severe cases of lumbar scoliosis or thoracolumbar scoliosis can degenerate and become lateral listhesis. Thoracolumbar curves have the greatest propensity for developing lateral listhesis during adulthood. Back pain may be more notable in severe thoracolumbar curves.

Just how common is this type of vertebral slippage? Who is prone to this destabilizing spinal complication of adult scoliosis?

Researchers in 2011[18] found that scoliosis with sideways slippage of the vertebrae was significantly more prevalent in women. They found that this problem typically only starts to occur after the age of 50, but will steadily increase with age. By the time the patients in the study were over 80 years old, nearly a quarter of them had the slippage.

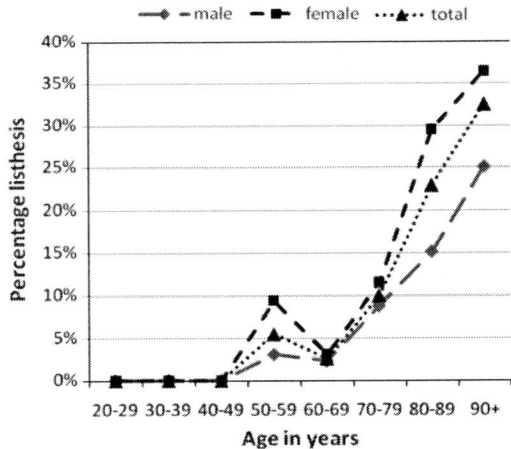

"As the adult lumbar spine ages, the prevalence of lateral listhesis and degenerative scoliosis increases."

---

18 Kilshaw M, Baker RP, Gardner R, Charosky S, Harding I. "Abnormalities of the lumbar spine in the coronal plane on plain abdominal radiographs." *European Spine Journal.* 2011 Mar;20(3):429-33. https://www.ncbi.nlm.nih.gov/pubmed/21069544

"In patients with a scoliosis 44 percent had a listhesis and in patients with no scoliosis just 3.8 percent had listhesis."

When we see a worsening of adult scoliosis, intervention with scoliosis-specific exercises is an effective treatment, not just to get stability, but to recover some degree of the postural collapse. This improvement of the scoliosis **does not** indicate a reduction of the degenerative changes, but instead indicates improvement of the upright posture which had begun to collapse. This improvement can decrease the chronic postural imbalance on the spine and, in the long run, reduce the risks of progression.

Corrective bracing can be a valuable tool to defeat postural collapse associated with laterolisthesis. The brace is put on while the patient is lying on their back. This position allows the maximal relaxation of the spinal muscles. Now the brace is tightened up and that less stressed posture is held by the brace. Adults typically wear the brace only six hours per day.

Degenerative Spondylolisthesis

Degenerative Spondylolisthesis occurs when a pre-existing forward misalignment causes the upper vertebra to slide forward on the lower vertebra and the tendons, muscles and the ligaments yield under the pressure, leading to ligament instability. Degenerative Spondylolisthesis is not always associated with spondylolysis.

The degree of spondylolisthesis is measured according to the **Taillard index**:

Grade 0	No slipping
Grade I	Minimal slipping of less than 1/3 of the width of the bones
Grade II	Slipping of 1/3 to 2/3 of the width of the bones
Grade III	Slipping of more than 2/3 of the width of the bones
Grade IV	Spondyloptosis: a complete slip, past the front edge of the lower vertebra. This condition is often associated with spinal cord compression (cauda equina syndrome (latin for "horse's tail") or central stenosis).

Let's look at some more research into the risk of degenerative slippage in the spine.

Risk of Progression (small curves)

In one study, VERY SMALL CURVES were studied. Even in this group of very small curves (only an average of 14 degrees at the beginning of the study), curve progression was found in de novo degenerative scoliotic curves.

"46 percent of patients had lateral listhesis of more than 5 mm at L3 and L4. Curve progression was not linear and might occur rapidly, particularly in women older than 69 with lateral listhesis of more than 5 mm and levoscoliosis."

Loss of Height and Slippage of the Vertebrae

"Average shrinkage in scoliotic women was twice that in the non-scoliotic women, had begun early in adulthood, was due to the combined effect of age and scoliosis, and was strongly associated with rotatory olisthesis. In the 17 women with radiograph follow-up, curve progression was closely related to shrinkage."

Surgery vs Conservative Treatment

One study[19] found a significantly higher rate of spinal stenosis and degenerative spondylolisthesis in patients who underwent surgery (decompression and spondylodesis).

---

19 Kluba T, Dikmenli G, Dietz K, Giehl JP, Niemeyer T. "Comparison of surgical and conservative treatment for degenerative lumbar scoliosis." *Archives of Orthopedic Trauma Surgery.* 2009 Jan;129(1):1-5. https://www.ncbi.nlm.nih.gov/pubmed/18560848

Chapter 10. Scoliosis and Osteoporosis

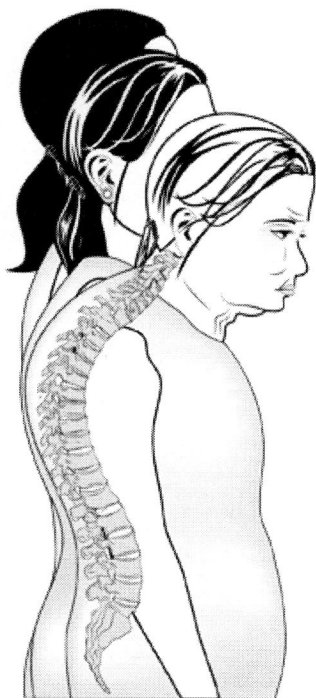

A concern with degenerative or adult-onset scoliosis is how it is affected by osteoporosis. Osteoporosis and scoliosis are related because they are both conditions which affect the spine. Osteoporosis is a disease that affects the density or mass of bone structures. Millions are diagnosed with the condition, which decreases the strength of bone and may lead to reduced protection against fractures. It is accompanied by brittle and/or porous bones and is associated with loss of bone-building nutrients such as calcium, vitamin D and magnesium.

Osteoporosis by itself isn't associated with pain, but compression fractures that may result because of it can be very painful. About 15-20 million people have osteoporosis, and over half a million out of this group suffer spinal fractures due to osteoporosis each year.

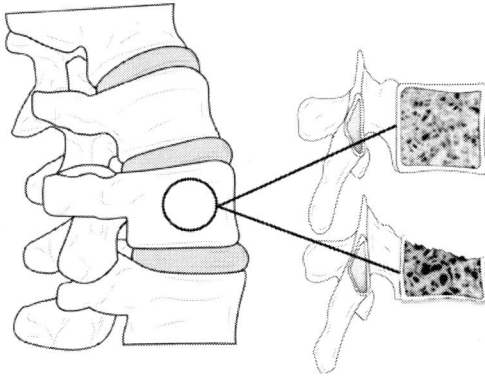

Image above shows loss of bone matrix associated with osteoporosis.

While osteoporosis does not cause scoliosis, it is highly associated with it. This means that the two conditions are commonly found together. It is very important for young people with scoliosis to understand the relationship of scoliosis and osteoporosis and begin calcium and vitamin D supplementation at an early age. Due to vertebral fracture, osteoporosis can also cause kyphosis or a rounded or humped back

Risk Factors for Osteoporosis

Gender

Women are at a greater risk of developing osteoporosis because they generally have less bone mass than men. Also, hormonal changes that take place during menopause can deplete bone density, and women tend to live longer than men. Though women are at greater risk, roughly 2 million men in the U.S. have osteoporosis and another 3 million are at risk.

Genetics

Asian and Caucasian women who are small boned, are at highest risk for osteoporosis. Similarly, there is a greater tendency for Adolescent Idiopathic Scoliosis patients to be slender females. This connection has stimulated scientists to look into the connection and studies have suggested a possible link between scoliosis and osteoporosis. One study states that osteopenia (bone density that is lower than normal) is common among AIS patients and "The prevalence of osteoporosis in AIS patients is much higher than in the general pediatric and adolescent population"[20]. This prevalence carries over to Adults with Adolescent Idiopathic Scoliosis.

Like scoliosis, osteoporosis runs in families. Though family history increases your risk of developing the condition, it does not mean you WILL develop it. A study investigating the link between scoliosis and osteoporosis compared **body mass index (BMI)** and **bone mass density (BMD)** of AIS patients to that of their siblings. The study found that not only did the patients with scoliosis have lower BMIs, but they also had lower bone masses than their siblings with normal spines[21]. This suggests a connection between the two disorders. The details of the connection are still to be determined. Does scoliosis cause osteoporosis? Does osteoporosis cause scoliosis?

Lifestyle

Certain lifestyle choices have also been linked to osteoporosis. Poor diet, smoking, excessive consumption of alcohol, and inactivity can all increase your risk.

Other Conditions

Certain metabolic disorders can also contribute to osteoporosis such as Cushing's syndrome, hyperthyroidism, and hyperparathyroidism. As well as certain gastrointestinal disorders that can affect the body's ability to absorb calcium.

Preventing Osteoporosis

Supplements

After the age of 18, all women (particularly postmenopausal women) are advised to take calcium along with vitamin D. Talk to your doctor to determine which calcium and what amount is appropriate for you.

---

20 Xin-Feng Li, Hai Li, Zu-De Liu, Li-Yang Dai. "Low bone mineral status in adolescent idiopathic scoliosis." *European Spine Journal.* 2008 Nov;17(11):1431–1440. https://www.ncbi.nlm.nih.gov/pmc/articles/PMC2583185/

21 Sadat-Ali M, Al-Othman A, Bubshait D, Al-Dakheel D. "Does scoliosis causes low bone mass? A comparative study between siblings." *European Spine Journal.* 2008 Jul;17(7):944–947. https://www.ncbi.nlm.nih.gov/pmc/articles/PMC2443267/

Diet & Exercise

Staying in shape through moderate exercise is also advisable for prevention of many conditions and diseases including osteoporosis.

With osteoporosis and adult scoliosis, precaution must be observed before exercising. These conditions offer different challenges depending on age, severity and prognosis. It is best to discuss with a scoliosis exercise specialist which types of exercise are best for your specific case and which should be avoided. Specialized exercise recommendations for adult scoliosis patients are based on health history, physical examination, and x-ray results.

Exercise that maintains or increases flexibility may be beneficial if you've been diagnosed with osteoporosis and scoliosis. Low-impact and gentle stretching and toning exercises such as yoga, Pilates, and tai chi may reduce pain and improve the limited range of motion caused by either condition. Walking is another low-impact, weight-bearing exercise that helps maintain flexibility, strength, and stamina.

Cautions

If you've been diagnosed with low bone mass or osteoporosis, talk to your scoliosis professional about safe exercises that won't worsen your condition or cause further injury to bones and joints. Avoid high-impact exercises that severely affect the bones and joints.

Back pain is the most common symptom of this condition, and x-rays may show wedge or compression fractures of the vertebrae. It is very important to confirm a diagnosis of osteoporosis as symptoms occur with other conditions such as infections, other metabolic bone diseases, and benign or malignant bone tumors. The extent of the osteoporosis can only be estimated on X-rays and must be confirmed by specific bone density tests or, in some cases, by bone biopsy.

CALCIUM TYPES & ABSORBTION

CHARACTERISTICS IN ORDER OF VALUE IN HUMAN NUTRITION

	ADVANTAGES	DISADVANTAGES
1 MICROCRYSTALLINE HYDROXYAPATITE 24% CA	• Best absorbed calcium source • Increases cortical bone density • Arrests trabecular bone loss • Absorbed by malabsorbers • Proven by scientific studies on humans	• None
2 CITRATE 22% CA	• Very well absorbed • Reduces risk to kidney stones • Absorbed by those with poor digestion	• Poor uptake into bone • Urinated out quickly
3 ASPARATE 10% CA	• Well absorbed	• Expensive
4 ASCORBATE 10% CA	• Well absorbed • Non-Acidic Vitamin C (neutral ph-well tolerated)	• Expensive
5 LACTATE 18% CA	• Well absorbed	• May contain milk and/or Yeast by-product, Source - fermentation of molasses, Starch, sugar or whey with calcium carbonate.
6 AMINOACID CHELATE 20% CA	• Well absorbed	• Soy Sensitivity • Often incorrectly made • Sometimes blend is not a true chelate
7 PHOSPHATE 29% CA	• Inexpensive • Antacid	• Fair absorption • Possible lead content from phosphate rock
8 CALCIUM CARBONATE 40% CA	• Inexpensive	• Poorly absorbed

Types of calcium supplements. Hydroxyapatite is the winner.

Chapter 11. Pregnancy and Scoliosis

Will Scoliosis Interfere with My Fertility or Ability to Carry a Baby to Term?

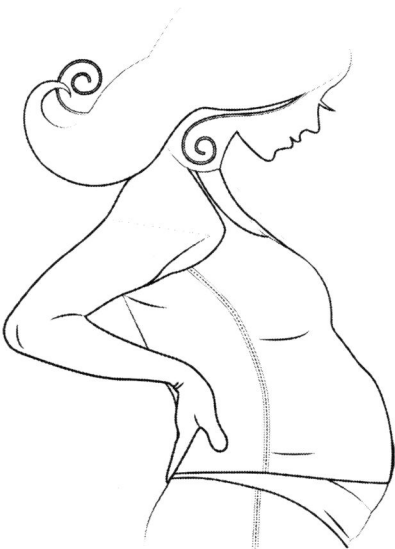

Since idiopathic scoliosis in adults is common in women of childbearing age, there are concerns about the effects it may have on pregnancy or becoming pregnant. Over the past 40 years, several studies have been conducted with hundreds of women who showed **NO** difference in pregnancy, labor, delivery, and fetal complications – whether they had scoliosis or not.

There is **NO** evidence that scoliosis reduces fertility or leads to an increased number of miscarriages, stillbirths, or congenital malformations.

Scoliosis does not have an adverse effect on becoming pregnant or the ability to deliver full-term children – even in large-curve cases.

What About Pregnancy Potentially Causing Rapid Progression of the Curve?

Another major pregnancy concern is increased risk of progression of the scoliosis. Some studies[22] have shown that patients lost 2, 6 and 18 degrees of correction during their first pregnancies, but curves stayed the same or improved with later pregnancies. So, while there can be a time of curve progression during the first pregnancy, this research concluded that generally scoliosis does not increase during a woman's subsequent pregnancies. As long as the curve is not in a progressive phase, the weight gained during pregnancy does not trigger an increase in the scoliotic curvature.

Just to confuse things, a review of the literature completed in 2011 by Schroeder and Dettori[23] found that pregnancy does not appear to affect curve progression. However, the editors of the journal make a point that the evidence was of a low quality. This was because the review was on all kinds of scoliosis, not just the types discussed in this book. Also, the data was obviously on adults, but the baseline comparison was on data about adolescents. Not a good match! The last issue was that the literature review only looked at curve size and did not look at other issues that adults are concerned about, like pain levels or percentage of patients who had surgery.

Lebel and Sergienko[24] studied modes of delivery and pregnancy outcomes for patients with scoliosis. They found that scoliosis is not a risk factor for problem deliveries.

Aside from a mild degree of restricted lung capacity, individuals with mild to moderate size idiopathic scoliosis rarely experience breathing problems during pregnancy, unless there is a pre-existing lung condition or im-

---

22 Blount WP, Mellencamp D. "The effect of pregnancy on idiopathic scoliosis." —NCBI. 1980. https://www.ncbi.nlm.nih.gov/pubmed/7430194

23 Schroeder, J.,Dettori,JR, Ecker,E, and Kaplan, L." Does pregnancy increase curve progression in women with scoliosis treated without surgery?" *Evidence-Based Spine-Care Journal.* 2011 Aug; 2(3): 43–50. https://www.ncbi.nlm.nih.gov/pmc/articles/PMC3604750/

24 Journal of Maternity Fetal and Neonatal Medicine 2012 Jun;25(6):631-41.

pairment. Breathlessness on exertion is a common complaint in the early months of pregnancy for all women (with or without scoliosis).

Shortness of breath is partly caused by the rise in progesterone, which stimulates breathing by increasing respiratory rate and the depth of each breath. Blood volume also increases. These normal physiological changes are well-tolerated and only likely to be problematic if the vital capacity is low or heart function is compromised. A very large scoliosis that occurs in the middle spine may affect breathing. Bladder and bowel problems may be an issue for women with scoliosis who already have urinary or bowel dysfunction.

Back Pain and Scoliosis During Pregnancy

Physical health and pre-existing back problems can affect the amount of back pain experienced when pregnant. It's been stated that as many as 40 percent of women who have had their scoliosis surgically corrected experience increased low back pain during pregnancy.[25] However, many women with no abnormal curvature still have mild to moderate back pain during pregnancy, so it can be difficult to distinguish whether the pain is from the scoliosis or pregnancy. Maintaining a good fitness program and addressing existing back problems prior to pregnancy may help mothers avoid or reduce back discomfort.

Pregnancy Back Pain Management

Specific treatment and rehabilitation for scoliosis is especially important throughout pregnancy for reducing weakness and back or neck pain. This type of back pain can be treated by targeting the specific area of concern. Acute treatment in conjunction with ergonomic adaptation and a specific program of lower back exercises designed for each scoliosis patient can decrease stress on the lower back and alleviate pain.

---

25 Orvomaa, E. "Pregnancy and Delivery in Patients Operated by the ... – NCBI." 1997. 26 Apr. 2016 http://www.ncbi.nlm.nih.gov/pubmed/9391799

Some other activities can be practiced for pain relief. Ice or cold compresses can help. Some pain in the muscles can be alleviated with warm compresses or by sitting in a warm tub or jacuzzi (NOT TOO HOT/100° F). Maternity support belts can be worn that support the lower back and stomach, allowing freer movement. Swimming is also great exercise during pregnancy, as the water will help support the stomach and also allow for freer movement. Strengthening exercises, such as pelvic-tilt exercises can help strengthen the back and relieve pain–always consult your doctor before initiating any exercise program.

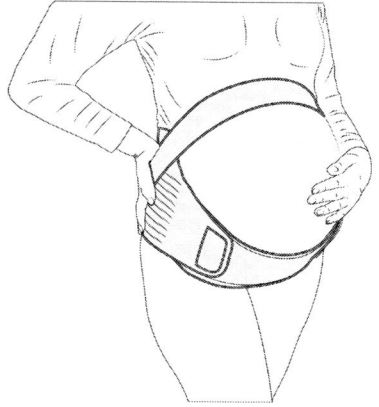

Pelvic-tilt Exercises

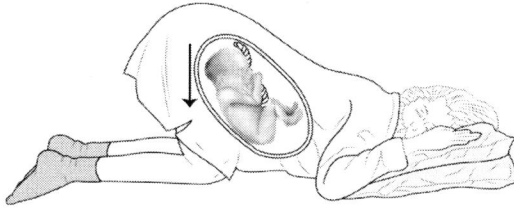

Often, just putting yourself into the knee-chest position to move the baby out of the pelvis and off of your pelvic nerves may make you more comfortable.

Knee-chest Position

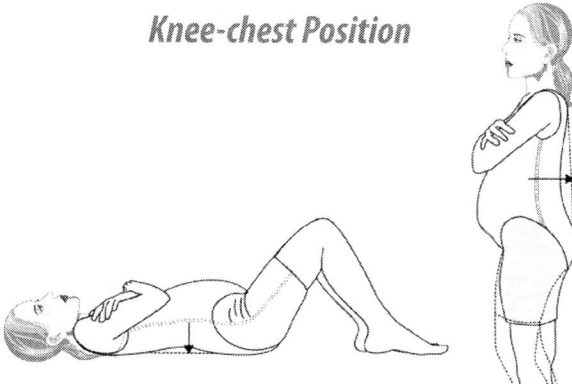

Pregnancy and Severe Scoliosis

Women with very severe scoliosis (over an 80-degree Cobb angle) should consult their obstetrician before becoming pregnant, as some cases may require monitoring of the scoliosis and fetus. Also, because the uterus pushes the diaphragm higher and decreases capacity, some breathing problems may be experienced during the later stages of pregnancy. Health-care providers may choose to manage these respiratory problems by prescribing non-invasive positive pressure ventilation through a CPAP. Back pain can also be significant for pregnant women with severe scoliosis, compared to non-scoliotic patients.

Labor & Delivery

If you are thinking of having an epidural, make sure to consult with your anesthesiologist well before your delivery date. Explain to the doctor that you have scoliosis and be sure tolet him see an X-ray of your spine. The epidural is inserted between the lumbar vertebrae and if you have significant rotation in the lumbar spine, the doctor responsible for your epidural will need to account for the change in needle insertion for his pain control planning.

Pregnancy and Congenital Scoliosis

Individuals with congenital scoliosis or early-onset scoliosis and those with weak muscles and heart problems should seek medical advice before becoming pregnant. Congenital scoliosis is often associated with neuromuscular conditions such as muscular dystrophy or poliomyelitis. These are genetic, and some can be detected prenatally.

Breathing will also be affected if the muscles that expand the rib cage are weak. Lung size may also be more severely restricted because of certain birth defects. Evidence suggests that as long as the vital capacity exceeds around 1.25 liters, the outcome will probably be good. Below this level, problems with a reduction in oxygen worsen on exertion and during sleep and may be accompanied by a rise in carbon dioxide levels. Low oxygen levels are harmful for the growing baby and also can lead to heart strain in the mother. CPAP ventilation machines have been used to guard the health of mothers and facilitate the birth of healthy, full-term babies.[26]

To ensure a healthy pregnancy, scoliosis patients need to follow the guidelines for proper nutrition, rest, exercise, prenatal medical, and chiropractic care as outlined by their obstetricians. Patients also should see their scoliosis specialists regularly to monitor curve status.

26 Allred, CC. "Successful Use of Noninvasive Ventilation in Pregnancy." 2014. 25 Apr. 2016 http://err.ersjournals.com/content/23/131/142.full.pdf

> *Three passions, simple but overwhelmingly strong, have governed my life: the longing for love, the search for knowledge, and unbearable pity for the suffering of mankind.*
>
> – **Bertrand Russell**

Chapter 12. Relieving Scoliosis Pain

I Thought Scoliosis Wasn't Painful!

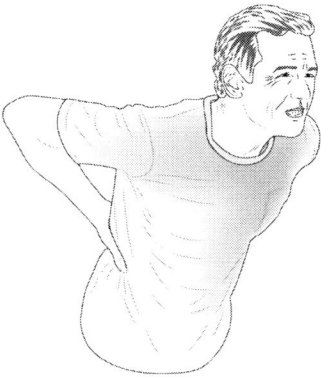

The absence of any strong pain associated with scoliosis is an identifying hallmark of a diagnosis of infantile, juvenile, and adolescent idiopathic scoliosis. In children, the presence of significant pain is considered an important clinical indicator that the scoliosis may be a symptom of some underlying issue such as a pinched nerve, tumors, infection, disc herniation, spinal cysts, scars, abdominal muscle spasms, or muscle and ligament damage due to traumatic injury. However, mild to moderate pain is often present in children with scoliosis and strong pain can be an all too common finding of adult scoliosis.

Is Scoliosis Causing My Back Pain?

Pain is often a common problem reported by adults with either adult degenerative\de-novo scoliosis (DDS) or adolescent scoliosis in an adult (ASA). Activity-related musculoskeletal pain is much more common in adults with scoliosis. As the adult spine undergoes degenerative changes, water content in the discs is reduced and this predisposes the spine to inflammation. Nerve impingement or "pinched nerves" may occur as a result of a spinal misalignment. Other sources of pain are arthritis of the facet joints, disc bulges, and disc herniations.

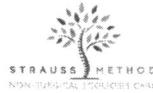

STRAUSS METHOD
NON-SURGICAL SCOLIOSIS CARE

• IN A 2007 STUDY •
OF 51 ADULT SCOLIOSIS SUFFERERS BETWEEN THE AGES OF 17 AND 60:

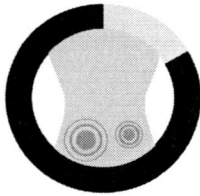

84%
(43 out of 51)
experienced low back
pain.

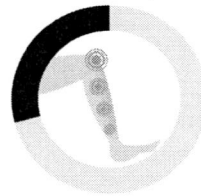

43%
(22 out of 51)
experienced nerve
root pain.

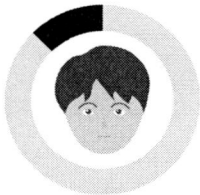

Only 8%
(4 out of 51) of patients
reported no pain at all.

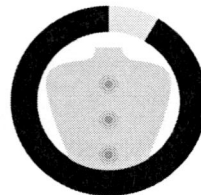

92%
of the sample group
said that they experi-
enced pain regularly
as a symptom of their
scoliosis.

Dr S. Kotwal from the world-renowned Hospital for Special Surgery in New York says that the clinical presentation of adult scoliosis is frequently associated with spine pain and neurogenic claudication.[27]

Neurogenic claudication in adult scoliosis patients is typically caused by spinal stenosis (a narrowing of the spinal canal – the space in the vertebrae which the spinal cord runs through) in the lumbar spine (lower back). Narrowing of the spinal canal results from wear and tear and arthritic changes in the lower back including: disc bulges, thickening of ligaments, and bone spurs along the spine. The narrowing of the holes through which the nerves pass can compress the nerve roots and cause pain, tingling, or cramping.

Neurogenic claudication pain is typically worse when standing and walking because the spinal canal naturally narrows in an upright posture, placing greater pressure on the nerve roots. This pain can typically be temporarily relieved by sitting or leaning forward because the spinal canal naturally expands a bit, relieving pressure on the nerve roots.

Kotwal discusses in his paper[28] the treatment options for adult scoliosis and concludes that the possible negative effects of surgery are large. His non-operative treatment recommendations include physical conditioning and exercise, pharmacological agents for pain control, and use of orthotics (bracing) and invasive modalities like epidural and facet injections.

What Can I Do About My Scoliosis Pain?

Scoliosis Exercise Programs

The deep core muscles of the spine are mostly controlled automatically by a group of sensors in the brain stem. The effect of uncoordinated function

---

27 Kotwal, S, Pumberger, M., Hughes, A., Girardi, F. Degenerative Scoliosis: A Review." HSS Journal (2011) 7: 257. https://doi.org/10.1007/s11420-011-9204-5.

28 Ibid.

between the shorter and longer spinal muscles and back pain is just now becoming understood.[29]

Similarly, one of the drivers of idiopathic scoliosis is suspected to be primarily an incoordination between the deep core muscles of the spine which is correlated with increased incidence of back pain.

Since most of the traditional therapeutic exercise programs for back pain focus on strength, endurance, fitness, and functional capacity only, the connection between idiopathic scoliosis and therapeutic exercise for back pain seemed remote. However, a new understanding of neuromuscular discoordination syndromes is starting to provide insight into the relationship between back pain and scoliosis pain.

A 2000 study highlights why "one size fits all" type therapeutic exercise for back pain associated with any structural problem and especially for patients with scoliosis is inappropriate.

"There is considerable variability in the nature and degree of the motor control problems presenting in patients with low back pain. In the future, links may be found between specific variables in the patterns of muscle control exhibited by patients with low back pain and the tendency for severity or persistence of the condition.

In the short term, this variability between patients highlights the need for an individual problem-solving approach to the neuromuscular dysfunction in patients with low back pain in the clinical situation." [30]

29 Dietz, V. "Proprioception and Locomotor Disorders – UFJF." 2002. 25 Apr. 2016 http://www.ufjf.br/especializacaofisioto/files/2013/06/Proprioception-and-loco-motor-disorders.pdf

30 Jull, GA. "Motor Control Problems in Patients with Spinal Pain: a New ..." 2000. 26 Apr. 2016 http://www.ncbi.nlm.nih.gov/pubmed/10714539

Why Do I Have More Pain in My Shoulder Than My Back?

Scoliosis and Shoulder Pain

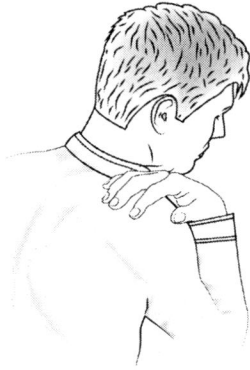

When shoulder pain develops, it will most often develop first on the shoulder on the side that the ribs are more prominent.

Therefore, if your spine curves to the right, you can expect the right shoulder to show signs of shoulder pain first. This is due to the tendons and muscles stretching as the body tries to overcompensate and pull the spine back into a normal position.

In addition, as scoliosis progresses without treatment, there is a risk that the opposite shoulder may begin to experience pain as it must endure increasing imbalance as the torso twists from the scoliosis. This leads to increased disability.

The pain in the shoulder region is expected and will continue without treatment.

An exercise-based scoliosis care program can effectively treat many of these types of shoulder pain by balancing the muscles, improving mobility, and most importantly guiding the spine back into a more central posture.

Scoliosis shoulder pain should be considered with all types of scoliosis as a potential health risk. Treatment is necessary to effectively prevent and decrease pain when the shoulders begin to feel the pull of the spinal curvature.

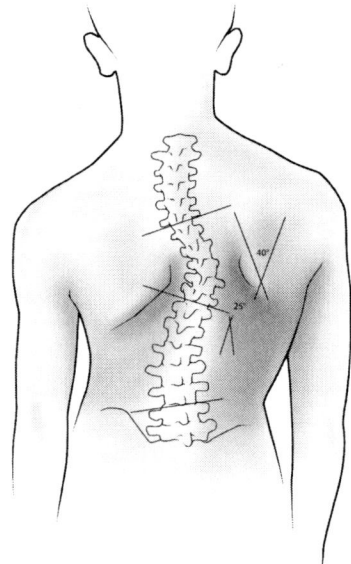

Scoliosis and Hip Pain

While less common than shoulder pain, many adults will experience pain in the hips associated with their scoliosis.

One of the identifying signs of scoliosis is having one side of the pelvic bones appear higher than the other. This can lead to pain when walking or standing for long periods of time. This is postural pain and is caused by the effects of gravity on the unbalanced posture. The wear and tear of unbalanced posture can lead to earlier than typical degenerative changes in the hip joints.

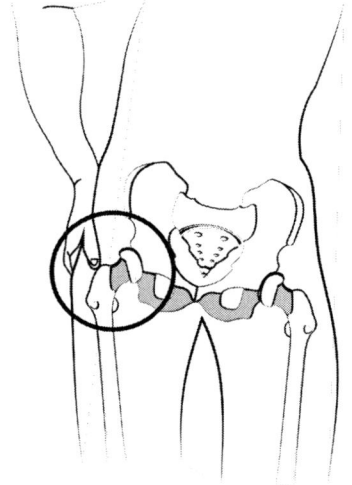

Also, if the pelvis is tilted from scoliosis, then one hip starts to take extra loading, eventually causing severe pain from the overuse/misuse of the tendons and musculature. The pain may subside with rest, but then returns. **Ligament laxity**, or looseness, can also cause pain and discomfort.

Sacroiliac Joint Pain

Sacroiliac (SI) joint dysfunction refers to pain in the sacroiliac joint region that is caused by too much or too little motion of the joint. This results in inflammation of the SI joint and can be debilitating. Scoliosis can trigger sacroiliac dysfunction because the weight of the body is shifted to one side, stressing the pelvic joints.

The pelvic girdle is made up of the iliac bones and the sacrum (tailbone). The sacrum connects on the right and left sides of the ilia (pelvic bones) to form the right and left sacroiliac joints.

Two major ligaments hold the joints together – the iliolumbar and sacroiliac ligaments. The **iliolumbar ligament** stretches from the top of the right and left iliac crest to its adjacent fourth and fifth lumbar vertebrae. The **sacro-**

iliac ligament stretches from the sacrum to its adjacent right and left iliac bones.

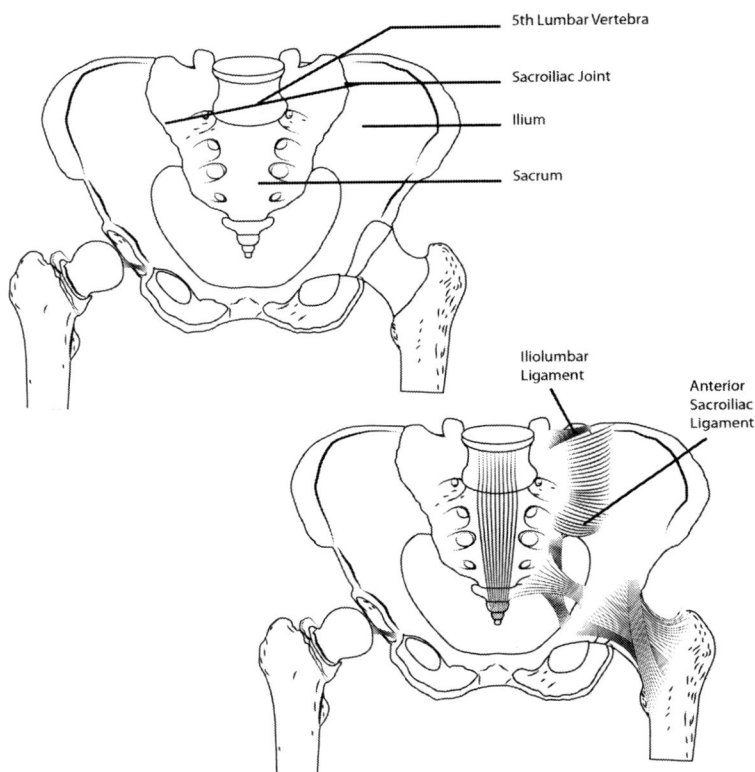

5th Lumbar Vertebra

Sacroiliac Joint

Ilium

Sacrum

Iliolumbar Ligament

Anterior Sacroiliac Ligament

The Many Causes of Sacroiliac Joint Pain

Strain and sprain of the iliolumbar ligament and sacroiliac ligament of the sacroiliac joint are common causes of low back, sacral, and other pelvic pain. Sprain to these ligaments is usually due to strain or traumatic injury (e.g. car accident, sports injury, fall). The abnormal postural strain of scoliosis creates long term stresses on the sacroiliac joints and often is an underlying cause of low back pain in the adult scoliosis patient.

Sacroiliac joint ligament sprain injuries are typically bilateral, meaning they affect both sides, though pain may be more pronounced on one side of the lower back. Lower back pain related to sacroiliac joint ligament sprain is commonly accompanied by misalignment of the sacroiliac joints and/or the lumbar vertebrae.

Sacroiliac Pain Symptoms

- Low back/groin/buttock/thigh pain

- Sciatica (pain down the back of the legs)

- Hip pain

- Increased urinary frequency

- Restricted mobility of the back and hips

- Difficulty walking or twisting

- Difficulty sitting or standing for extended periods

- Temporary numbness, prickling or tingling in the legs/feet

Low back pain from sacroiliac joint dysfunction can be isolated directly over the most problematic sacroiliac joint or both joints. Pain can range from dull aching to sharp and stabbing and will usually increase with physical activity.

Symptoms can worsen after holding prolonged positions (i.e., sitting, standing, lying down). Bending forward, climbing stairs, walking up a hill, and getting up from a seated position also can cause pain. Pain in the leg, groin, and hip is referred pain; the pain is felt in these areas instead of the site of the injury. Often, the pain of SIsprain injury spreads or projects in a shooting, radiating pain pattern that can be confused with "sciatica" or degenerative disc nerve root compression in the older patient. Severe and disabling sacroiliac joint dysfunction can cause insomnia.

Many muscles are connected with the ligaments of the sacroiliac joint including the piriformis. **Piriformis syndrome** is a condition often related to sacroiliac joint dysfunction. The piriformis muscle, located in the buttock region, spasms and causes pain in the buttock or even pain traveling down the leg that mimics sciatica.

Pain caused by this joint can refer in many different ways depending on the patient, because the nerves are interconnected. Severe and long-standing sacroiliac joint dysfunction can cause muscle deconditioning and atrophy throughout the body due to limitation of activities and exercise that cause low-back pain.

Leg Length Discrepancy Can Accompany SI Dysfunction

A functionally short leg accompanied by a slight limp and hip muscle weakness can be a sign of compensatory scoliosis or an accelerating force causing the scoliosis to become progressive. If your legs are two different lengths, a heel or full sole lift could correct the pelvic tilt and therefore ease some of the extra loading and alleviate some pain.

A 2006 study observed pelvic asymmetry associated with either C-type or S-type scoliosis and found apparent leg-length difference in 87 percent of the patients studied.[31]

Treatment

A sacroiliac belt may help reduce pain by stabilizing the sacroiliac joint to help maintain reduction of the misalignment and keep the joint in place between treatments.

The presence of a functionally short leg may require treatment with an orthotic device. If the short leg differential is less than 7-10 millimeters (mm), a heel lift rarely would be used, but a sole lift is needed when the discrepancy is over 10mm. In more extreme cases, the whole shoe may need to be built up by an orthotist.

---

31 Timgren, J. "Reversible Pelvic Asymmetry: an Overlooked ... – NCBI." 2006. 26 Apr. 2016 http://www.ncbi.nlm.nih.gov/pubmed/16949945

The amount of leg length shown on the X-ray can be misleading. Research shows that a specialized X ray known as the Fergusons View is needed to properly assess leg length. In addition, X-ray measurements are typically magnified by 25 percent due to the distance of the spine from the film (or X-ray sensor in a digital machine). This means that if the doctor measures 1 cm of leg length deficiency, the patient in reality has only a 7.5 mm deficiency.

Scoliosis and Stenosis

Each of the 33 bones of the spine have a large central opening for the spinal cord. Additional openings called the spinal foramen allow the nerves branching from the spinal cord to travel to the arms, legs and other parts of the body. **Foraminal stenosis** occurs when the neural foramen become drastically narrowed.

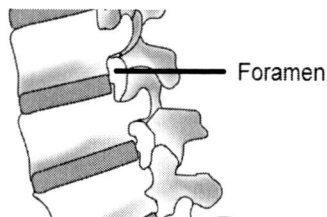

Foramen

Normally, nerve roots have enough room to easily slip through the foramen. However, with misalignment of the spine (subluxation) and conditions like arthritis, the foramen size may become reduced. Arthritic bony spurs can develop alongside the spinal openings and press on the nerves. This narrowing causes a restriction to the spinal canal, resulting in a neurological deficit. When the passage through which the spinal cord runs becomes narrowed, the condition is called **spinal stenosis.** The symptoms of spinal stenosis include pain, numbness, weakness, burning sensations, tingling and paraesthesia ("pins and needles") in the arms and legs, and loss of motor control.

Scoliosis and Sciatica

Sciatica and adult scoliosis can often coexist resulting in pain in the lower back and legs. Sciatica is a common form of pain that affects the sciatic nerve. The sciatic nerve extends from the lower back down through the back of each leg. Sciatica is caused by irritation or compression of the nerve roots of the lower spine. Sciatica can be caused by misaligned spinal bones (subluxation), lumbar spinal stenosis, and muscle spasm or piriformis syndrome (pain due to spasm in specific buttock muscles).

The symptoms of sciatica include:

• Pain in the buttocks or leg that worsens when sitting.

• Tingling or burning down the leg.

• Numbness, weakness, or difficulty moving the foot or leg.

• Constant pain on one side of the buttocks.

• Shooting pain making it difficult to stand up.

Sciatica commonly affects only one side of a person's lower body. Many times, the pain will extend from the person's lower back all the way through the back of their thigh and down through one of their legs. The pain the person experiences may also extend to one of their feet or into their toes, depending on how and where the sciatic nerve is irritated or compressed. The pain some people experience in relation to sciatica can be both severe and debilitating. Other people who experience sciatica find the associated pain to be infrequent and less irritating. Being overweight, not exercising regularly, wearing high heels, or sleeping on a mattress that is too soft may also make sciatica pain worse.

Can Scoliosis be the Cause of My Headaches?

Up to 50 percent of headaches can be attributed to neck problems. Chronic headaches are defined as occurring 15 days or more per month, for at least three months and lasting for more than four hours at a time (The Mayo Clinic). Chronic headaches

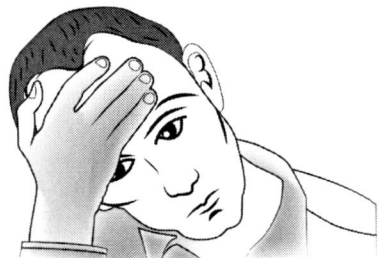

with neck pain usually involve a nerve pressure (subluxation) condition within the neck.[32]

Scoliosis can be associated with a muscle imbalance in the neck and shoulders, triggering headache. We discussed this earlier describing how there can be forward head position correlated with scoliosis and this can trigger headache.

Chronic Cervicogenic Headaches

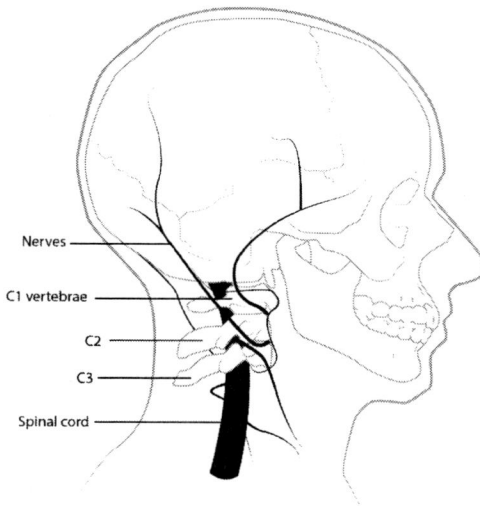

Nerves
C1 vertebrae
C2
C3
Spinal cord

There are seven vertebrae that make up the spine in the neck. These cervical vertebrae surround the spinal cord and canal. Between these vertebrae are discs, and the nerves of the neck pass nearby.

The top three cervical vertebrae are the most likely to refer pain to the back of the head and create a secondary type of headache, called a **cervicogenic headache**. Cervicogenic headaches are primarily occipital (at the base of the skull) head pain that originates and is referred from some joint, ligament, muscle, intervertebral disc and/or nerve in the upper neck. There is usually associated pain in the upper neck as well, which is frequently described as "dull," although the pain can become stabbing with head movement

32 Page, P. "Cervicogenic Headaches: An Evidence-led Approach ... – NCBI." 2011. 26 Apr. 2016 http://www.ncbi.nlm.nih.gov/pubmed/22034615

Causes of Cervicogenic Headaches

Trauma to the Neck

Muscles, ligaments, tendons, joints, discs and nerves of the upper neck can all be injured and cause neck pain, as well as headache. Whiplash from things such as falls, car accidents, or athletic injuries cause misalignments in the neck called or subluxations. Poor posture due to scoliosis can function as a low-level, but relentless micro-trauma to the neck. Any repetitive movements under this stress can cause subluxations, leading to neck pain and headaches.

Muscle Tension in the Neck

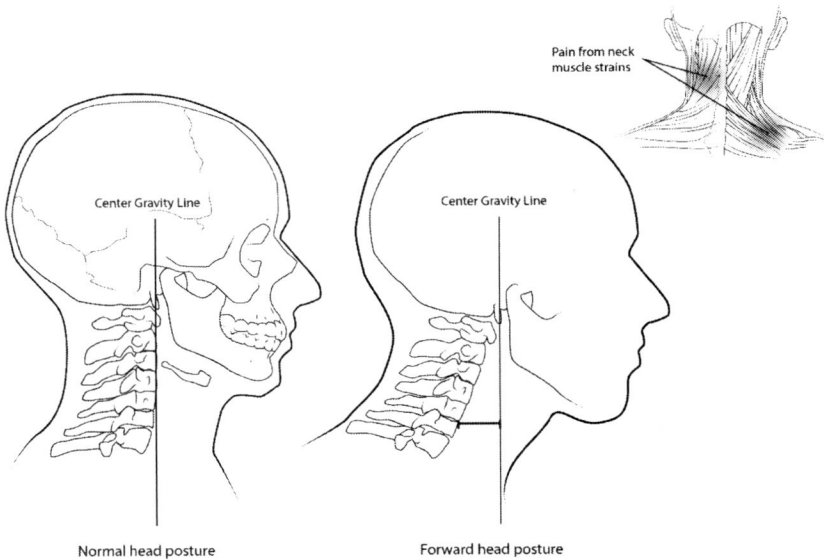

Pain from neck muscle strains

Center Gravity Line

Center Gravity Line

Normal head posture

Forward head posture

There are many muscles in the shoulders, neck and base of the head that can develop tension and inflammation and cause chronic neck and head pains. When neck and scalp muscles become tense and contract from stress, depression, a head injury, and/or anxiety, tension headaches can occur.

Scoliosis causes postural strain and often causes this type of neck muscle tension, which can lead to nerve pressure and tension headaches.

Tension headaches are the most common type of headache, and although a band-like constrictive pain around the head is most common, upper neck pain is not unusual. Computer work, stomach sleeping, and reading in bed also can trigger tension headaches.

Chapter 13. Scoliosis Assessment

What is the Doctor Looking for When He Examines Me?

We've established that watch-and-wait is a waste of critical time, but how should scoliosis be assessed and checked?

The evaluation of a patient should always begin with a comprehensive medical history and records review, a complete scoliosis examination (detailed below), and the appropriate X-rays. A comprehensive assessment should include:

Computerized postural assessment – A set of digital photographs are analyzed by computer software to precisely measure all postural distortions. This is used as a before-and-after evaluation tool. The photos will be from front, back and side.

Range of motion study – The doctor will ask you to move your spine gently through its complete range of motion to locate areas of restricted or excessive motion. This aids the doctor in understanding which area of the spine is most restricted, which curve is the "major," and identifies areas of pain more precisely.

X-ray evaluation – X-rays of the involved spinal areas will be taken. Special views will be taken if short leg syndrome or other abnormalities of the spine and pelvis are suspected. X-rays are crucial to secure an accurate analysis of the structure of the scoliosis. Dosage should always be reduced to the minimum possible.

Respiratory function assessment – This evaluation utilizes a computerized instrument that the patient blows into. Because certain scoliosis types can impact lung capacity, this test is vital for a full evaluation. If there is any lung involvement, corrective exercises can be prescribed or if the lung function is critically low, surgery may be indicated

Muscle strength and balance – The key muscles supporting the pelvis and the spine are evaluated for weakness and any side-to-side or front-to-back imbalance.

Coordination and proprioception – These areas are evaluated to determine the appropriate intensity for a custom-designed exercise program. The patient will be asked to balance on one foot, to march in place, and do other maneuvers to evaluate ability to perform home exercises. The program of scoliosis exercises must be individually designed to respect a patient's limitations. There is a link between poor balance and scoliosis, so this is a vital test. On the other hand, poor coordination and poor balance can be used in a positive way to make certain exercises like active self-correction more effective.

Scoliometer evaluation – This non-x-ray tool is used to approximate curve flexibility, size and location. The tool measures "angle of trunk rotation."

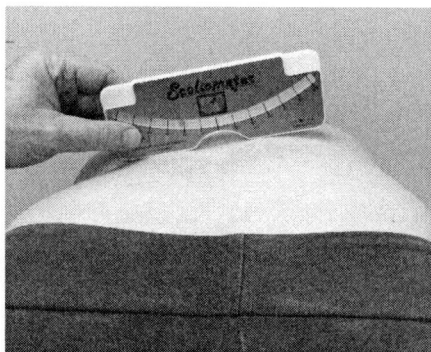

Spinal motion and static palpation – The doctor will move the spine gently to locate areas of inflammation and muscle tightness and to clarify location of restricted spinal segments.

Spinal cord tension testing – By determining the patient's flexibility and spinal cord length, the scoliosis specialist can prescribe appropriate stretching protocols. A relatively shortened spinal cord can be an underlying cause of scoliosis progression.

> *See my article, "Cord lengthening: Part of comprehensive AIS treatment", in Becker Spine Review for more detailed information: https://www.beckersspine.com/spine/item/37916-cord-lengthening-part-of-comprehensive-ais-treatment.html*

Foot evaluation – A computerized foot scanner will be used to identify and analyze excessive rolling of the foot (pronation or supination). While foot issues have never been shown to cause scoliosis, they are highly correlated with scoliosis. This means that they are often found in patients with scoliosis. Foot imbalances can impact stability of the spine and pelvis and are important to address. Leg length discrepancies may need addressing here too.

Biochemistry analysis – This test is used to evaluate for possible epigenetic (factors that can trigger genetic weaknesses to activate scoliosis progression), chemical, or hormonal scoliosis accelerators.

Pain scales – A questionnaire is used to analyze pain patterns. This before-and-after evaluation tool will help clarify symptomatic recovery.

Vitals – Vital data, including weight, blood pressure, and a very precise measurement of height are recorded. It is important to monitor height to see if a patient is increasing or decreasing in height.

Your scoliosis specialist will use this evaluation data to determine the best treatment plan to reduce or correct your scoliosis.

X-ray Safety

The amount of X-ray exposure the patient receives from X-ray evaluation is always a concern to both doctor and patient. This concern must be weighed against the importance of knowledge gained from the examination.

As humans we are continuously bombarded by radiation coming from natural sources. This radiation comes from outer space, the sun, the interior of the earth, radon gas, and other natural sources. The amount of radiation we get from natural sources varies depending on the elevation at which we live, how much time we spend in the sun, whether we live in a city or rural area, and our employment (think of an airplane crew spending many hours above the radiation protective ozone layer). Comparative study results show that the radiation from typical scoliosis X-rays is similar to a small fraction of the annual average exposure from natural sources.[33]

By using available X-ray-limiting technologies such as a high-frequency generator, digital capture, smaller film sizes, lead and aluminum foil shielding, and radiation reducing settings on the X-ray machine (high kV techniques), X-ray studies can be much safer and will expose the patient to significantly less radiation than standard full-spine films using conventional analog radiology.

New technologies have been developed to reduce radiation even further; however, at the time of the writing of this book, they are not deemed suitable for scoliosis evaluation except in extraordinary situations. A standing MRI allows for weight-bearing evaluation of scoliosis with zero radiation, but because of its high cost per evaluation, long scan time (3-4 minutes during which the patient must hold perfectly still... very difficult), and lack of standing MRI machines, this technology is not commonly used.

An ultra-low x-ray system called "EOS," or slit scan technology, has similar limitations because the scan is significantly more expensive and patients are

---

33 Pace, Nicola, Leonardo Ricci, and Stefano Negrini. "A Comparison Approach to Explain Risks Related to X-ray Imaging for Scoliosis, 2012 SOSORT Award Winner." *Scoliosis* 8.11 (2013): 7161-8. 19 Apr. 2016

subjected to longer times holding perfectly still. Raster stereography and Moire technology (also marketed as InSpeck, ISIS, Quantec and Frometric, which are based on the distortion which occurs when a grid of light is projected onto the back of the patient) hold great promise in analyzing scoliosis, but are not accurate enough to completely eliminate X-ray evaluation. Further research is needed in analyzing larger or obese patients and those with neuromuscular disorders.[34]

Radiation Exposure

While techniques vary from machine to machine and center to center, it is preferable for your scoliosis specialist to take "spot" view x-rays of the spine, which typically expose the patient to very little radiation. The 1 mSv (millisievert, a unit of measure) of radiation emitted during a spot x-ray registers an Additional Cancer Risk of 0.014378 percent, which is equal to 1 in 6,955 chances. (*Said another way, there is a 99.985622 percent chance of having no effect on the patient!*)

The chart below gives some perspective on radiation dosages by comparing the amount of radiation from various sources.

Comparison Doses			
Natural Background	3.1 mSv/year	**Domestic Pilots**	Additional 2.2 mSv/year
Average U.S. Total X-ray Exposure	6.2 mSv/year	**7-hour airline flight**	0.02 mSv
2 spot shot scoliosis views	0.1 mSv	**Chest CT Scan**	7.0 mSv

Ease Your Concerns

If you have concerns about your exposure to radiation or the type of x-rays being taken, discuss them with your scoliosis specialist.

---

34 Knott, Patrick et al. "SOSORT 2012 Consensus Paper: Reducing X-ray Exposure in Pediatric Patients with Scoliosis." *Scoliosis* 9.1 (2014): 1. 21 Apr. 2016

Ask your scoliosis specialist to provide lead shielding. There is a lead "shawl" which patients can wear during the x-rays that helps protect uninvolved areas of the body from x-ray exposure. An additional lead shielding is used to protect the breasts, testicles or ovaries and thyroid gland. In addition to shielding, there are specific machine settings that lower the effective dose. Obviously, no X-rays should be taken if a patient is either pregnant, actively trying to become pregnant, or just unsure if they are pregnant.

Is the damage due to low-dose radiation from medical imaging studies overstated? According to a group of eminent radiation scientists who published an article on the subject in the *American Journal of Clinical Oncology* in 2015, the answer is a very strong "YES"! Educate yourself further by Googling *"The Birth of the Illegitimate Linear No-threshold Model – An Invalid Paradigm for Estimating Risk Following Low-dose Radiation Exposure."* [35]

35 Siegel, JA. "The Birth of the Illegitimate Linear No-Threshold Model: An ..."
2015. 26 Apr. 2016 http://www.ncbi.nlm.nih.gov/pubmed/26535990

II. WHAT CAUSES THE TYPE OF SCOLIOSIS THAT STARTS IN CHILDHOOD?

Epigenetics and Idiopathic Scoliosis

Although considerable progress has been made in the past 25 years in understanding the underlying causes of idiopathic scoliosis, there still is no agreed-upon theory of cause.

The main problem with determining a single cause appears to be that idiopathic scoliosis does not result from one cause, but from multiple interacting factors along with a host of genetic predisposing factors.

To further complicate things, many researchers believe that there are two different and unique processes happening in scoliosis. First are the initiating processes, and second are the processes that cause curve progression. As the research unfolds there is increasing evidence of an underlying neurological disorder for idiopathic scoliosis.

Epigenetics, a relatively new science, is analyzing factors from the environment, disease, aging, and even normal development that stimulate the genetic expression of scoliosis.

> "Scientists have found the gene for shyness. They would have found it years ago, but it was hiding behind a couple of other genes."
>
> – Jonathan Katz

Chapter 14. Idiopathic Scoliosis and Genetics

Idiopathic scoliosis has been known to run in families. According to the University of Iowa Health Care department, a world leading scoliosis research facility, "Hereditary and congenital irregularities have emerged as the most probable causes of scoliosis today." Based on population studies, it is considered a single-gene disease with variable penetrance (the extent to which a particular gene or set of genes is expressed) and heterogeneity (the presence of a variety of genetic defects which cause the same disease).[36]

While genetics is believed to play a role in scoliosis, more than 80 percent of childhood scoliosis cases are deemed idiopathic, meaning the source of the condition is unknown. Despite the vast amount of research, the cause of idiopathic scoliosis remains unknown. It is possible scoliosis is inherited the way other genetic traits are passed down from parent to child. This theory is greatly supported by the frequency with which idiopathic scoliosis appears in families, co-occurring with parent, children, and siblings. Studies

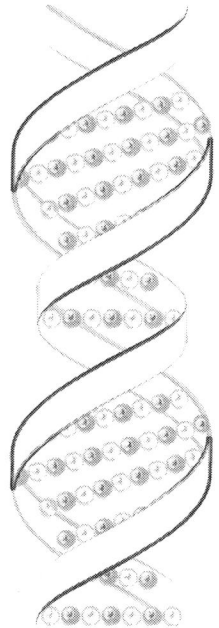

---

36 Tsiligiannis, T. "Pulmonary Function in Children with Idiopathic Scoliosis | Scoliosis and ..." 2012. 26 Apr. 2016 http://scoliosisjournal.biomedcentral.com/articles/10.1186/1748-7161-7-7

have shown the incidence of scoliosis in these cases is in the 7–11 percent range. In contrast, the incidence in grandparent, grandchild, uncle, aunt, nephew, niece, or half-sibling drops to less than 4 percent.

> **Factoid:** *Actress Isabella Rossellini and her daughter, model Elettra Wiedemann, both have scoliosis.*

In 2007, Texas Scottish Rite Hospital for Children researchers identified the first gene – CHD7 – associated with idiopathic scoliosis. It was the result of a 10-year study led by Carol Wise, Ph.D., conducted at the Sarah M. and Charles E. Seay/Martha and Pat Beard Center for Excellence in Spine Research. In 2011, they identified two additional genes – CHL1 and DSCAM – which play a role in the neurological and spinal systems. These findings will allow for new hypotheses for the etiology of scoliosis and serve as a tool for further research.[37]

Alain Moreau, Ph.D., head of the molecular genetics lab for musculoskeletal diseases at the Ste-Justine University Hospital Centre, Montréal, Canada said in an interview:

"Most likely, scoliosis is not a purely genetic disease. Although genetic factors are important, a 'cross talk' between genetics and some environmental factors is evident. The nature of these environmental factors, however, is unclear. The underlying genetic defects may be present at birth, but because the clinical manifestations usually occur at adolescence or prepubescence, scoliotic deformities must be triggered by environmental factors, which also include hormonal changes associated with puberty.

Increased levels of estrogen at puberty could explain why girls are more affected in number and severity than boys. Blood tests can now identify children at

---

37 "Genetic Scoliosis Research – Texas Scottish Rite Hospital ..." 2013. 15 Apr. 2016
http://www.tsrhc.org/genetic-scoliosis-research

risk of developing scoliosis. We need to do more work on phenotype and trying to make sense of that and correlating it to genotype."[38]

So, while genes may play a key role, like other genetic conditions, environmental factors may influence or even bring out this genetic predisposition. More genetic research and discoveries will fuel better understanding of the causes of scoliosis – specifically idiopathic scoliosis. Genetic research may provide the answer for what causes scoliosis, and it also may lead to improved preventive measures and treatment.

38 "Gene CHD7 Linked with Scoliosis [Archive] – National ..." 2009. 15 Apr. 2016
http://www.scoliosis.org/forum/archive/index.php/t-8938.html

> *The environment is everything that isn't me.*
>
> – **Albert Einstein**

Chapter 15. Does Scoliosis Have Environmental Triggers?

It is believed that many people carry genes that trigger the development and/or progression of scoliosis. The genetics may or may not be "expressed," and the person may or may not develop scoliosis. Experts largely agree that a variety of genetic variations at the chromosomal level predispose a person to a condition like scoliosis. These genetic variants need to be activated or "turned on" by something.[39] That "something" has been studied intensely, and has been widely reported on in the scientific literature. Research concludes that there are a wide variety of influencers. These "triggers" range from ONE OR EVEN SEVERAL of the following partial list:

1. Abnormal development of the front of the spinal bones.

2. Unsynchronized growth between the spinal column and the spinal cord.

3. Instability in the spinal joints due to loss of normal curvatures. which should be seen from a side view.

4. Spinal joint disorders which are made worse by the twisted spinal bones like arthritis and disc herniations.

5. Poor sensorimotor integration.

6. Motor control disorder.

---

39 Burwell, R Geoffrey et al. "Whither the Etiopathogenesis (and Scoliogeny) of Adolescent Idiopathic Scoliosis? Incorporating Presentations on Scoliogeny at the 2012 IRSSD and SRS Meetings." *Scoliosis* 8.1 (2013): 4. 21 Apr. 2016

7. Deformations of the spinal joints from birth defects.

8. Sensory integration disorder.

9. Disorders of neurodevelopment.

10. Defects in specific hormone receptors.

11. Protein signaling defects.

12. Maternal age at birth.

13. Infants using heated indoor swimming pools.

14. Body composition imbalances like obesity.

15. Exposure to specific bacteria (mycobacteria).

16. Metabolism disorders including abnormalities of:

    a) Platelet calmodulin

    b) Melatonin

    c) Melatonin signaling defect

    d) Osteopontin

    e) Oestrogens

    f) Leptin

    g) Bone calcium (osteopenia and osteoporosis)

17. Biomechanical misalignments of the spine and pelvis.

18. Balance disorders.

19. Body spatial disorientation.

20. Trauma (e.g. sports injuries, car accidents, occupational stresses, slips and falls).

21. Postural stress (e.g. slouching, sitting at work or school, driving a car, or even the postural stress of standing with an imbalanced spine).

22. Nutritional deficiencies and or excesses.

23. Aging.

Scoliosis and Nutrition

The impact that nutrition plays as an environmental influence on idiopathic scoliosis is poorly understood. Researchers consider nutrition as a minor contributing factor in the progression of adult scoliosis. While dietary changes are emphatically NOT the only care a scoliosis patient requires, let's take a look at what scientific studies are finding about the link between nutrition and scoliosis.

We know that poor nutrition can lead to many diseases, deformities, and conditions. For example, though there is no single cause of spina bifida nor a known way to prevent it entirely, folic acid taken before and during pregnancy has been shown to reduce its incidence. Rickets, the most common childhood disease in developing countries, is bone softening attributed to a deficiency or impaired metabolism of vitamin D, phosphorus, or calcium, potentially leading to fractures and deformity. Though it can occur in adults, the majority of cases occur in children suffering from severe malnutrition from famine or starvation during early childhood. Osteomalacia, a similar condition occurring in adults, is also generally due to a deficiency of vitamin D.

Could dietary deficiencies be a factor in the triggering or progression of adult idiopathic and/or de novo scoliosis? Researchers in one US study looked at articles from American and European journals, conference proceedings, and relevant research from 1955-1990 and found strong evidence (from animal studies) that poor nutrition could be a contributing factor in idiopathic scoliosis. While acknowledging limited human study data, they noted enough anecdotal evidence to warrant further investigation into a possible link between poor nutrition and the cause of Idiopathic scoliosis.[40]

---

40 Worthington, V. "Nutrition as an Environmental Factor in the Etiology of ... – NCBI." 1993. 26 Apr. 2016. http://www.ncbi.nlm.nih.gov/pubmed/8492060

Other research shows a possible correlation between too much copper and incidence of childhood scoliosis. Copper, an essential nutritional mineral, is involved in energy production and the formation of red blood cells, bone, and hemoglobin. It is also essential to nerve health, building and maintaining myelin, the insulating sheath that surrounds nerve cells. Copper aids an enzyme involved in the production of collagen and elastin, two connective tissue proteins. Copper also works with zinc and vitamin C to form elastin. It's necessary for the development and the maintenance of skin, bones, blood vessels, and joints, but can be problematic if elevated.[41]

Specific Mineral Function Has Been Studied in Children with Idiopathic Scoliosis

A 2008 study from Czechia (Czech Republic) showed the changes of selenium, copper, and zinc content in hair and serum of patients with idiopathic scoliosis. The patients studied were age 13 on average and had idiopathic scoliosis curves ranging between 12 and 82 degrees. The hair of these patients showed significantly increased zinc and copper (Cu) content and decreased selenium (Se) content when compared with the control group. The Cu/Se ratio in this group of patients was significantly higher due to a higher Cu value and a lower Se value in comparison with the controls. Also, compared with the controls, the serum selenium concentration in the group of scoliotic patients was significantly decreased.[42]

A 2002 study from Czechia on idiopathic scoliosis and concentrations of zinc, copper, selenium, albumin, and ceruloplasmin in blood and the activity of superoxide dismutase plasma found a significant decrease of selenium when compared with a control group. The same levels of significance were found for selenium levels corrected for albumin content.

In a group of patients with a curvature over 45 degrees (medically this size curve is often recommended for surgical intervention) the average plasma

41 Burwell, RG. "Adolescent Idiopathic Scoliosis (AIS), Environment..." 2011. 25 Apr. 2016. http://scoliosisjournal.biomedcentral.com/articles/10.1186/1748-7161-6-26

42 Dastych, M. "Changes of Selenium, Copper, and Zinc Content in Hair and ..." 2008. http://www.ncbi.nlm.nih.gov/pubmed/18404661 25 Apr. 2016.

concentrations of selenium were significantly lower in comparison with a group of patients with a curvature below 45 degrees who were treated conservatively.

The decreased concentration of selenium in the blood plasma suggests possible negative effects on the process of synthesis and maturation of collagen affecting axial skeleton (i.e, skull, spine, ribs) stability.[43]

Just to show that there is no consensus on selenium, an article from China says the opposite, stating high selenium levels are linked as a risk factor for developing scoliosis!

Nearly 10,000 cases from three areas in China were included in this study. Each region had different selenium levels.

Researchers found high selenium levels significantly associated with AIS development, whereas low selenium levels had no significant correlation with AIS development. They also found that females in the high selenium group had larger curves than males. These results align with typical male/female presentation seen with idiopathic scoliosis.

This study suggests that high selenium content is one of risk factors for adolescent idiopathic scoliosis. The authors of the study suggest that very high selenium levels may not cause scoliosis as the symptoms of selenium poisoning do not include scoliosis. However, a large number of animal experiments suggested that ingesting a certain amount of selenium would significantly boost body development. They suggest that the "growth-promoting effect of selenium" resulted in spinal overgrowth during the growth cycle and led to scoliosis. But this hypothesis was still inconsistent with some phenomena during investigation. [44]

---

43 Dastych, M. "Idiopathic Scoliosis and Concentrations of Zinc ... – NCBI." 2002. http://www.ncbi.nlm.nih.gov/pubmed/12449234 25 Apr. 2016.

44 Ji, X et al. "Change of Selenium in Environment and Risk of Adolescent Idiopathic Scoliosis: a Retrospective Cohort Study." *Eur Rev Med Pharmacol Sci* 17.18 (2013): 2499-503. 21 Apr. 2016.

As indicated at the beginning of this article, idiopathic scoliosis is most likely caused by a genetic predisposition brought out by some external force. Some research suggests a link between nutrition and AIS, but this is probably an effect of a genetic defect rather than a cause. Perhaps the gene(s) responsible for scoliosis are also responsible for the malabsorption/retention of certain nutrients in the scoliotic patient. In other words, it may not be that the patient has poor eating habits, but that they have a biological inability to store or remove certain nutrients in their body.

Idiopathic scoliosis is associated with whole organism metabolic phenomena, including:

- lower body mass index

- lower circulating leptin levels

- other systemic disorders (those which affect multiple parts or the whole body).[45]

---

45 Burwell, RG. "Scoliogeny of Adolescent Idiopathic Scoliosis: Inviting ..." 2013. 25 Apr. 2016. http://scoliosisjournal.biomedcentral.com/articles/10.1186/ 1748-7161-8-8

> *"The internal machinery of life, the chemistry of the parts, is something beautiful. And it turns out that all life is interconnected with all other life."*
>
> **– Richard P. Feynman**

Chapter 16. The Hormone-Scoliosis Connection

Let's take a step back in time to explore the frequent onset of scoliosis during one of the most important hormonal based changes in a person's life – adolescence. Using that understanding, let's then look at de novo scoliosis that accelerates during the other important time of hormonal change – menopause.

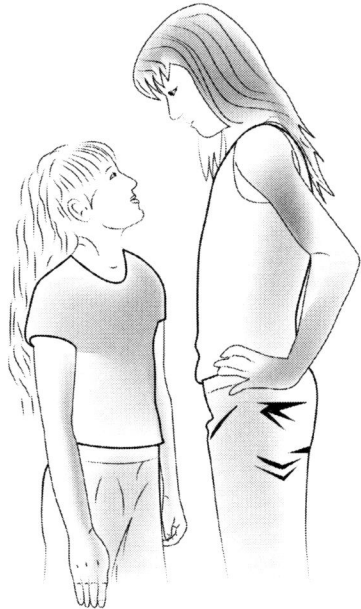

Studies suggest that one of the catalysts for the manifestation of adolescent idiopathic, as well as postmenopausal de novo scoliosis, may involve a significant change in estrogen levels, the hormones that triggers the onset of puberty as well as menopause.

There is already plenty of research that supports a multifactorial cause of scoliosis and (as we've previously mentioned) the involvement of genetic and epigenetic predispositions and the influence of hormonal factors are also widely accepted. Adolescent idiopathic scoliosis is assumed to be associated with a sex-linked predominant gene with incomplete penetrance (meaning that symptoms are not always present in individuals who have the genetic mutation) and variable expression (meaning variations in type and severity of a genetic disorder can exist between individuals with the same genetic mutation, even within the same family).

There are twice as many girls than boys with Cobb angles greater than 10 degrees and eight times as many with Cobb angles greater than 30 degrees. Are hormones the only reason AIS occurs more frequently in girls than boys? A study from 2012 illustrates how adolescent idiopathic scoliosis occurs 2-10 times more frequently in females than in males. This observation is postulated to be due to the **Carter effect.** (Males are more likely to transmit the disease to their children, but not have AIS themselves.) In this situation males would need to inherit a greater number of susceptibility genes compared to females to develop AIS and would also be more likely to transmit the disease to their children and to have siblings with AIS. In the families they tested, AIS was lowest in sons of affected mothers (36 percent) and highest in daughters of affected fathers (85 percent). Affected fathers transmitted AIS to 80 percent of the children in the test, whereas affected mothers transmitted it to 56 percent. Siblings of affected males also had a significantly higher prevalence of AIS (55 percent) compared with siblings of affected females (45 percent). Researchers state that the presence of the Carter effect supports the multifactorial threshold model of inheritance in AIS.[46]

What Role Might Estrogen Have in Scoliosis Formation?

It is believed that AIS develops in two stages: **1)** initial functional impairment of osteoblasts and osteoclasts (which control the amount of bone tissue: osteoblasts form bone, osteoclasts repair/remodel bone), and **2)** the stage of actual spinal deformation. However, the reason is still unknown.

Estrogens have a modifying influence on bone growth and remodeling, and control changes in the structure of cancellous bones (spongy bone).

---

46 Kruse, LM. "Polygenic Threshold Model with Sex Dimorphism in ... – NCBI." 2012. 26 Apr. 2016. http://www.ncbi.nlm.nih.gov/pubmed/22992817

The research is not suggesting that estrogens cause AIS, but that due to their function, they may affect progression. Menopause is the natural decline in reproductive hormones. This typically occurs when a woman is between 45 and 55 years old. Estrogen deficiency is associated with increased bone turnover, increased osteoclast activity and increased osteoblast activity. Estrogens also regulate the activity of melatonin receptors and inhibit the synthesis of melatonin. They interact with other hormones and biochemical factors, such as calcium-binding protein calmodulin, as well as with other proteins controlling muscle contractility.

"Understanding the role of estrogens seems vital for explaining the evolution of AIS associated with skeletal growth..." [47]

47 Kulis, Aleksandra et al. "Participation of Sex Hormones in Multifactorial Pathogenesis of Adolescent Idiopathic Scoliosis." *International Orthopaedics* 39.6 (2015): 1227-1236. 19 Apr. 2016.

Chapter 17. How Do Normal Daily Activities Affect Scoliosis?

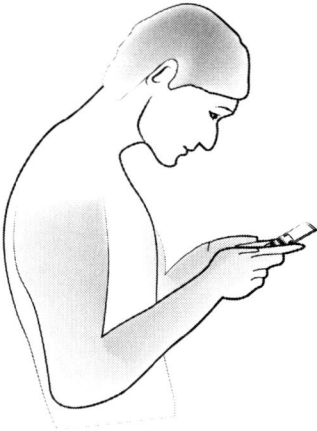

Typical daily activities are also known as "Activities of Daily Living" (ADLs). These are the activities that people do routinely every day.

We all know that improper posture, both standing and seated, is bad for the joints and especially bad for the back, but could it be worse for adults with scoliosis? Research suggests that while poor posture cannot "cause" scoliosis, poor posture can exacerbate scoliosis. Specifically, increased time spent in an improper seated position can lead to asymmetry of the spine and the back.

A study published in 2014 examined the effects of seated position on children age 11 to 13. Researchers found that extended periods of sitting caused a flattening of the normal and healthy curve of the middle back.[48] If results like these can be found with young, healthy spines, what might the research show when studying older test subjects?

Slouching! This has been suggested as a risk factor leading to the expression of scoliosis. This may not come as a shock, given the amount of time we sit

---

48 Drza-Grabiec, J. "Effects of the Sitting Position on the Body Posture of ... – NCBI." 2015. 26 Apr. 2016. http://www.ncbi.nlm.nih.gov/pubmed/24962297

at work, in a car or bus, and in front of a TV or computer. As technology advances and life becomes more automated, we can stay seated for longer periods.

A study published in 2008 looked at the amount of time people in the United States spend in sedentary activities. They found the most inactive groups are older adolescents (16–19 years) and older adults (60 years and older).

"Given the large amount of time spent each day in sedentary behaviors in the United States, efforts to reduce the amount of time spent in low-energy-expenditure pursuits are warranted."[49]

Is Sitting the Only Issue? What About Other Activities?

Sitting is an issue, but let's look a little closer at other activities common to daily living.

Ergonomics is the scientific study of how people interact with their environment and how to eliminate injuries or disorders that can develop from repetitive movements, bad posture, and overuse of muscles. Businesses capitalize on findings by designing ergonomic furniture and products to make movements easier and to prevent injury.[50]

Modifications to **activities of daily living** (ADLs) at home, during exercise or at work can make a huge difference in posture.

How you sit in a chair matters, particularly if you are in it for hours on end. How you carry a tote or purse affects posture, too.

---

49 Saunders, Travis J, Jean-Philippe Chaput, and Mark S Tremblay. "Sedentary Behaviour as an Emerging Risk Factor for Cardiometabolic Diseases in Children and Youth." *Canadian Journal of Diabetes* 38.1 (2014): 53-61. Print.

50 "CDC – Ergonomics and Musculoskeletal Disorders – NIOSH ..." 2003. 20 Apr. 2016 http://www.cdc.gov/niosh/topics/ergonomics/

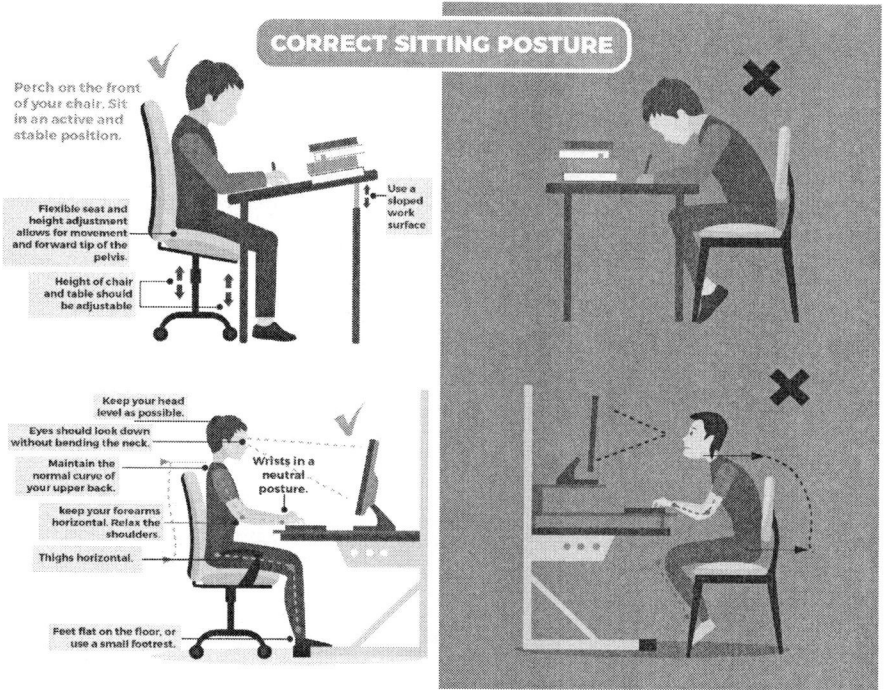

Have you ever noticed that it's easier to carry a purse or messenger bag on one shoulder than on the other side? Why is that?

Does carrying a heavy purse or briefcase cause permanent damage? What kind of damage could it cause?

The adjacent image depicts the effect of carrying a bag on one shoulder. Notice how the body naturally leans in the opposite direction to compensate for the added weight.

Now imagine that this person already has a spinal curvature toward the right. It is possible to modify how you carry your backpack, purse or groceries to help manage scoliosis.

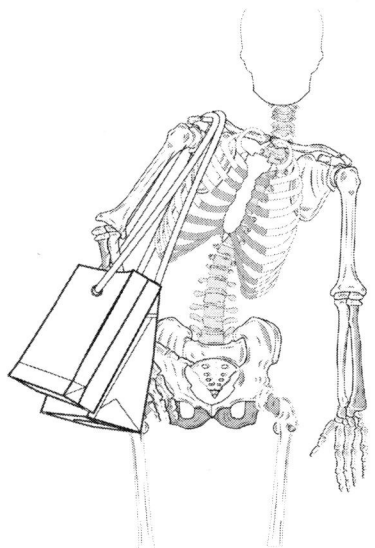

The use of external aids can also help with your treatment program. These aids can include:

- **Prism glasses** – to hold the head upright while texting and playing games on the phone or tablet.

- **Heel, sole or ischial lifts** – to balance any leg or pelvic asymmetry like a leg length deficiency.

- **Orthotics** – used along with stable footwear to minimize the effects of pronation on the spine. While pronation does not cause scoliosis, the pelvic instability associated with significant pronation can work to destabilize corrections achieved by other aspects of a scoliosis specific home exercise program.

A single session of ergonomic intervention can show significant improvement in seated posture. Reduction of handbag or briefcase weight helps too. Proper ergonomics (office seating along with proper positioning of the computer monitor, keyboard and mouse) can impact scoliosis-care programs in a positive way.

Patients are always asking me what they can do outside of their scoliosis treatment program to help reduce pain or encourage their curve reduction. I have developed a program to assess what comprises patients' daily activities and what modifications can benefit their spinal curvatures. I have presented this at an advanced scoliosis conference, and now many scoliosis clinicians are helping their patients with simple modifications to their normal everyday activities.

Applying the principles of active self-correction; sitting, standing, and walking can be modified to greatly assist in stabilizing the curves of the adult with scoliosis. It is not possible in a book to advise the method of correction because each scoliosis is unique in a variety of ways, and this individuality must be taken into consideration in the design of the active self-correction program.

Active Self Correction forms the foundation of most scoliosis-specific exercise programs. This type of exercise must be done during the patient's normal daily activities. These maneuvers are different from other forms of exercise because they are meant to be performed continuously throughout the day. The exercises are performed by the patient without any external assistance in the form of props or instruction from a therapist.

The idea of the self-corrective maneuvers is to place the spine in a scoliosis-reduced posture. While a therapist is used along with various props during the training period, the patient must ultimately be able to perform the maneuvers alone without any props. The patient is instructed to attempt to hold the corrected posture as much as possible during their day.

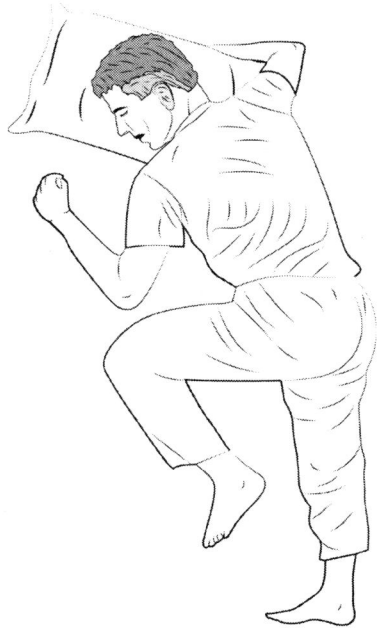

During sleep. the patient is instructed to use rolls, cushions, and wedges to place the body in a stable somewhat de-rotated position. This encourages the development of the normal spinal contours and also works to de-rotate the pelvis and rib cage. While the patient may not be able to maintain this position all night, if they can place themselves in a de-rotated posture for at least 20 minutes as they go off to sleep, it is therapeutic and will assist in their spinal correction and stabilization.

> *Education is the most powerful weapon which you can use to change the world.*
>
> **– Nelson Mandela**

III. SCOLIOSIS TREATMENT

Chapter 18. Bizarre Historical Scoliosis Treatments

The existence of scoliosis in humans is likely as old as the existence of man. There is a long history of its presentation from King Tutankhamun to Hippocrates. Because of this, there is a vast and fascinating history of both the condition and its treatment. Interestingly, many of the bygone forms of treatment are very similar to today's treatments.

An article published in the 2009 *Scoliosis Journal* details the history of spinal deformities and their treatment. In Ancient Greece "medicine" was practiced at Asclepions, temples dedicated to Aesculapius, the god of health. A priest-physician conducted treatments such as hydrotherapy, physiotherapy, hygienic rule, diet, drug therapies and minor surgical procedures. (Figure 1)[51]

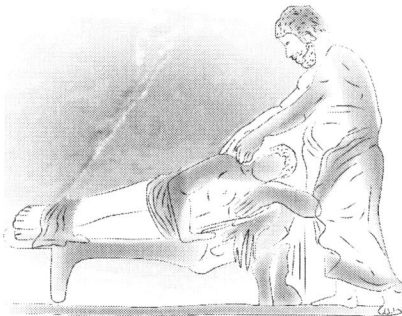

Figure 1. Aesculapius, the god of health, examines a patient.

51 Vasiliadis, ES. "Historical Overview of Spinal Deformities in Ancient Greece ..." 2009. 26 Apr. 2016. http://scoliosisjournal.biomedcentral.com/articles/10.1186/1748-7161-4-6

The authors suggest that such practices were most likely also used to treat spinal deformities.

Hippocrates (460-370 B.C.) recommended diet and extension for the treatment of scoliosis. During the time of Hippocrates, spinal manipulation was widely used as a treatment for scoliosis; however, he was the first to invent devices based on principles of stretching and lengthening the spine, as well as how to apply corrective pressure to straighten spinal curvatures. Hippocratic books do not contain illustrations of these techniques but Apollonius of Kitium (first century B.C.) wrote of Hippocrates techniques in On *Articulations*, and illustrations were found in a Florentine surgical manuscript, Laurentianus (ninth century A.D.) (Figures 2, 3 and 5).

Hippocratic Ladder

The Hippocratic ladder was developed to reduce spinal curvatures. To achieve reduction, the patient was shaken while tied on a ladder – in an erect position if the rib arch was near the neck or with the head downward if the rib arch was at a lower level. Body weight pulled and straightened the spine. Hippocrates described the board as the most efficient method for the correction of spinal deformities because the physician could easily control the forces exercised on the spine and those forces were exerted naturally (Figure 2).

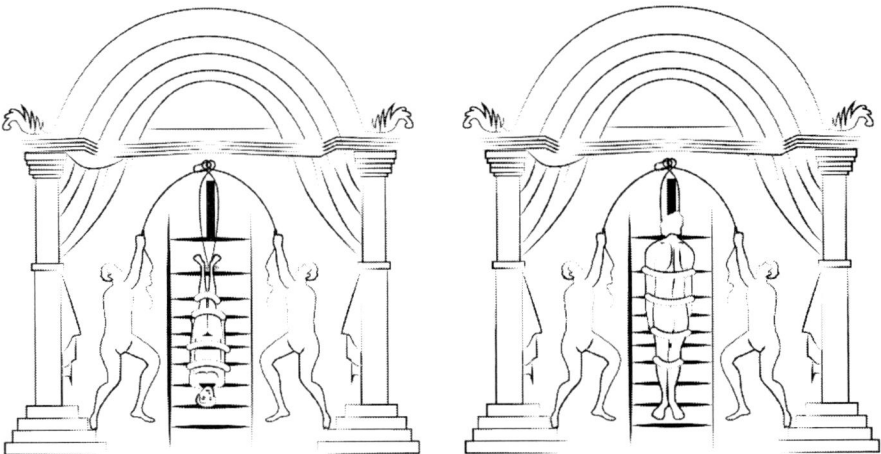

Figure 2. Hippocratic Ladder.

Hippocratic Board

The Hippocratic Board is another device to manage spinal curvatures. Simultaneous traction of the spine and the manual application of focal pressure over the kyphotic area was recommended:

"But the physicians, or some person who is strong, and not uninstructed, should apply the palm of the hand to the hump, and then, having laid the other hand upon the former, he should make pressure, attending whether this force should be applied directly downward, or toward the head, or toward the hips ... and there is nothing to prevent a person from placing a foot on the hump, and supporting his weight on it, and making gentle pressure; one of the men who is practiced in the palestra[52]* would be a proper person for doing this in a suitable manner."* (Figures 3 and 4).

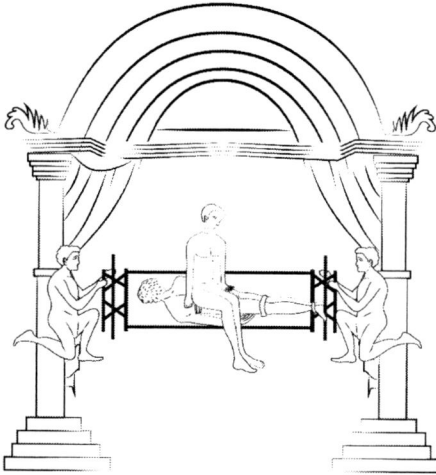

Figure 3. Hippocratic board.

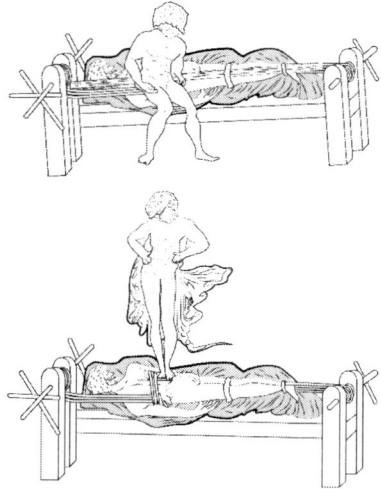

Figure 4. Correction of spinal deformity with the Hippocratic board.

52 * A public place in ancient Greece for training and practice in wrestling and other athletics.

For patients requiring stronger forces, Hippocrates recommended:

"The apparatus for forcible reduction should be arranged as follows. One may fix in the ground a strong broad plank having in it a transverse groove. Or, instead of the plank, one may cut a transverse groove in a wall, a cubit above the ground, or as may be convenient. Then place a sort of quadrangular oak board parallel with the wall and far enough from it that one may pass between if necessary; and spread cloaks on the board, or something that shall be soft, but not very yielding...." (Figure 5)

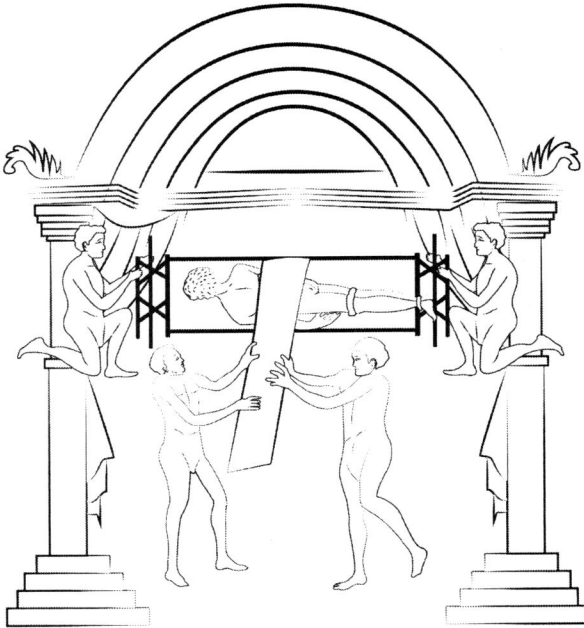

Figure 5. Hippocratic board used with a plank on the hump.

"...A soft band, sufficiently broad and long, composed of two strands, should be applied at its middle to the middle of the chest, and passed twice round it as near as possible to the armpits; then let what remains of the (two) bands be passed round the shoulders at each side, and the ends be attached to a pestle-shaped pole, adjusting their length to that of the underlying board against which the pestle-shaped pole is put, using it as a fulcrum to make extension." (Figure 6).

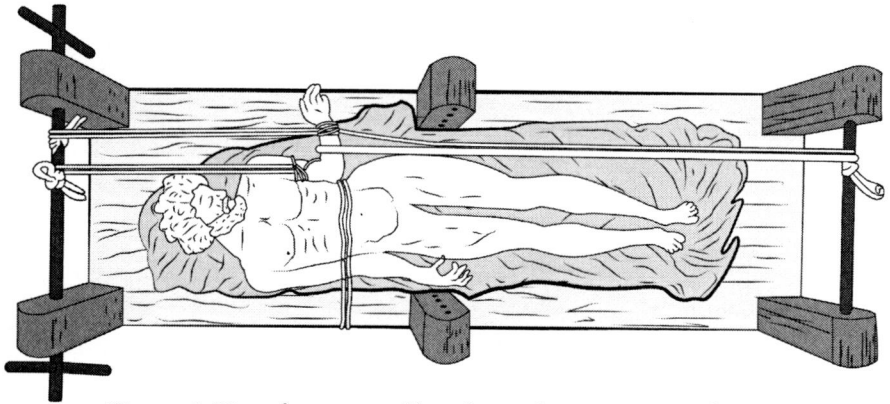

Figure 6. Use of straps and bands on the Hippocratic board.

Oribasius (325-400 A.D.), a Byzantine physician, modified the Hippocratic board by adding a bar. He used it for gradual reduction of both spinal traumas and deformities. (Figure 7).

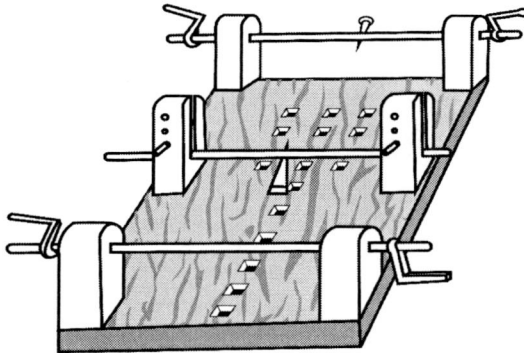

Figure 7. A third bar was added to the Hippocratic board.

Hippocratic Scamnum

The third device for the management of spinal deformities was the Hippocratic scamnum (Figure 8):

"But the most powerful of the mechanical means is this; if the hole in the wall, or in the piece of wood fastened into the ground, be made as much below the man's back as may be judged proper, and if a board, made of lime-tree, or any wood, and not too narrow, be put into the hole, then a rag, folded several times

or a small leather cushion, should be laid on the hump ... when matters are thus adjusted, one person, or two if necessary, must press down at the end of the board, while others at the same time make extension and counter-extension along the body, as formerly described."

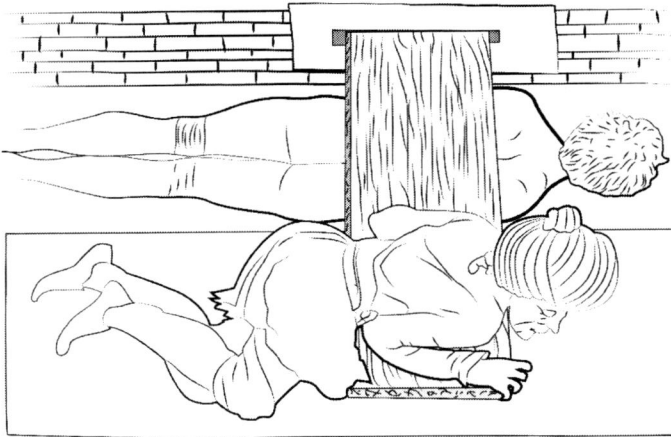

Figure 8. The Hippocratic scamnum.

Galen (129–216 A.D.) recommended the use of the Hippocratic board (Figure 9) for traumatic deformities and the Hippocratic ladder for kyphotic deformities, although he expressed his doubts on the effectiveness of this technique.

Paulus of Aegina (625–690 A.D.) lived during the Byzantine period, but is still considered the last physician of Greek antiquity. He used the Hippocratic board for management of spinal deformities and also emphasized it in the use of orthoses in spinal trauma and deformities.[53] Controversy surrounded the next methods I am going to describe. These protocols were used in France as early as 1820, documents show.

---

53 Vasiliadis, ES. "Historical Overview of Spinal Deformities in Ancient Greece ..." 2009. 26 Apr. 2016. http://scoliosisjournal.biomedcentral.com/articles/10.1186/1748-7161-4-6

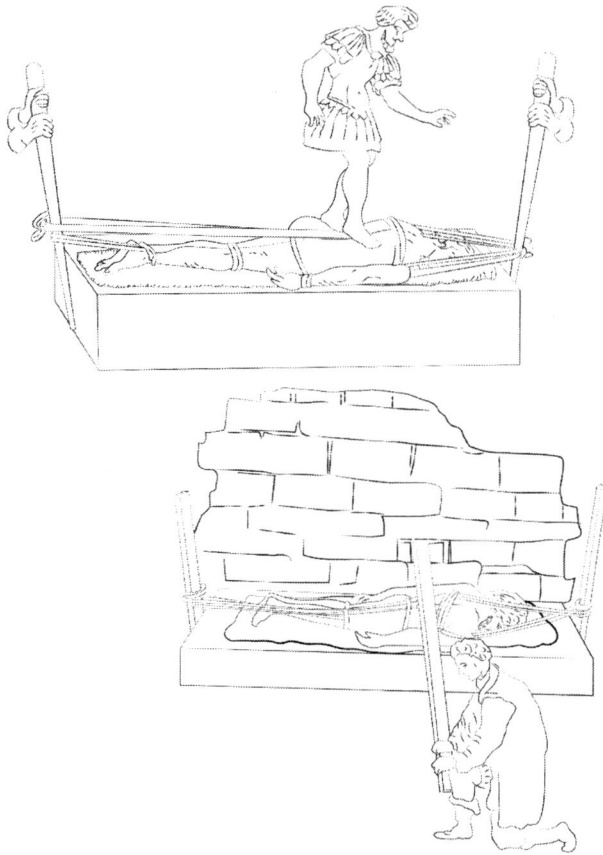

Figure 9. Galen's devices were similar to the Hippocratic board and scamnum.

At the time, surgeons were using powerful mechanical means to perform traction on the spinal column to correct deformity, which in some cases led to paralysis. The Royal Academy of Medicine was involved and certain practices were discredited.

Surgeons set up a research society to monitor the complications. As recently as 1975, the research society reported an incidence of paralysis of 0.72 percent (57 cases!) in a sample of 7885 patients. There were many causes, but excessive traction on the spinal column most definitely caused preventable paralysis. The transmitted force on the spinal cord and the nerve roots would have been tremendous once surgeons cut stabilizing ligaments. Paralysis also resulted when forcible traction was applied by halo – even without dividing the ligaments.

In 1764, Francois Guillaume Levacher de la Feutrie introduced the first mechanical bed in France. The bed was designed to "push on the bumps" in an attempt to cure rickets. It only was used on children because of their soft adaptable bones It would have been used periodically for up to two weeks at a time, applying gentle pressure. The bed did not exert traction on both extremities of the body, therefore avoiding adverse effects (Figures 10 and 11).

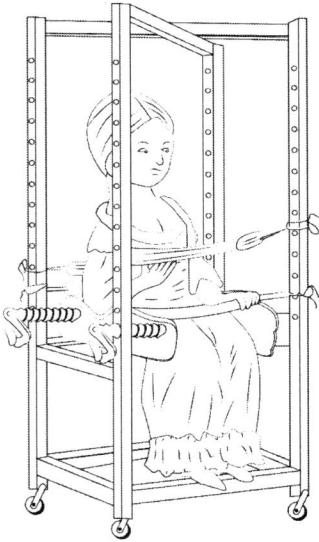

Figure 10. Extension chair by Levacher.

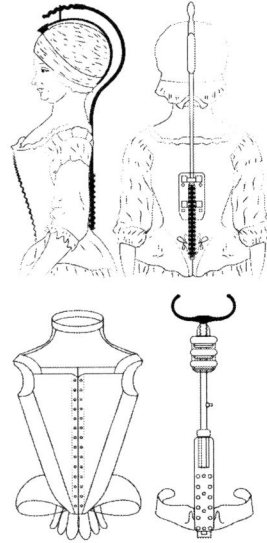

Figure 11. Minerva jacket by Levacher.

Charles Gabriel Pravaz (1791-1853) believed scoliosis resulted from unequal growth or activity. His extension equipment allowed patients to remain in an upright position as he was a critic of the previously designed horizontal beds. He emphasized the importance for patients to self-adjust the traction. Pravaz used gentle traction therapy for no more than two hours a day with no adverse effects (Figure 12).

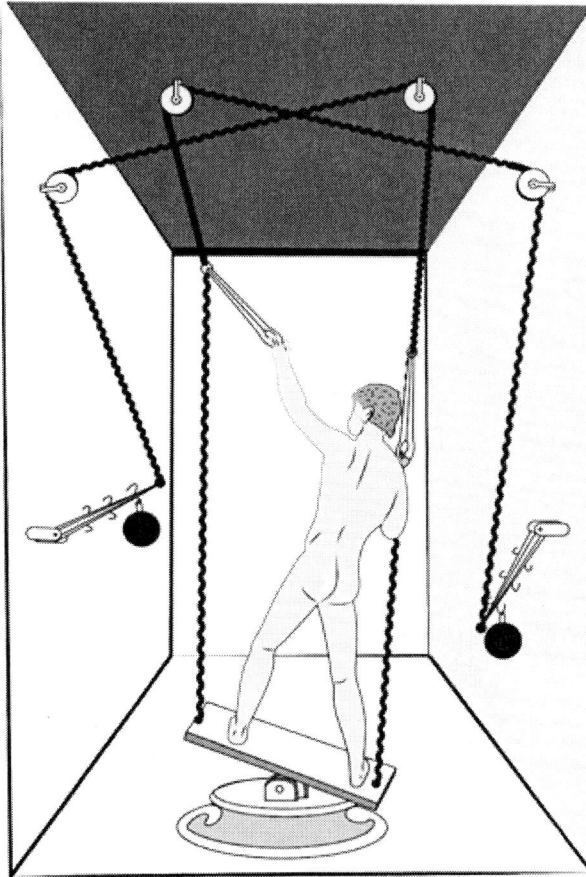

Figure 12. Balançoire Othopédique by Pravaz.

In the 1820s, Charles-Auguste Maisonabe introduced his version of the mechanical bed, which used weights attached to straps or ropes that were tied to the patient's pelvis and head. It used very strong traction. The bed also was equipped with a dialed scale to gauge how far weights had moved from the applied force. Maisonabe was unable to measure the resistance of the spinal column, and therefore found it very difficult to gauge the amount of weight required. His solution was to pull the patient's head manually to estimate the weights required for each patient and to err on the side of caution. One would increase tension by shortening the straps or ropes (Figure 13).

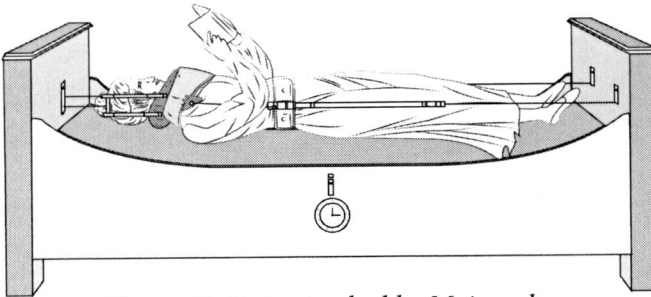

Figure 13. Extension bed by Maisonabe.

Many doctors were strongly against the use of extension beds, causing much controversy at the time. Some even accused proponents of "self-interest and poor physiological knowledge."[54]

Ambrose Paré, a famous French army surgeon, is considered the father of modern surgery and treatment with prostheses and supportive orthotic devices. He developed the first scoliosis brace in the 16th century. It was made of iron plates (Figure 14). The brace was further developed in the 18th and 19th centuries in France and Germany (Figure 15).

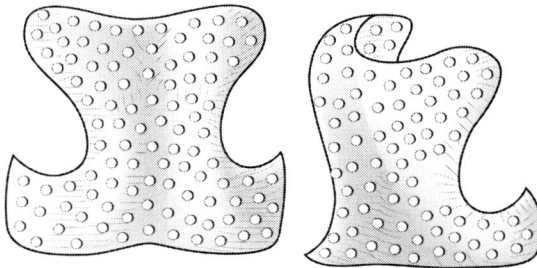

Figure 14. First support metal braces by Paré.

54 Weiner, MF. "Abstract – Nature Publishing Group." 2009. 26 Apr. 2016. http://www.nature.com/sc/journal/v47/n6/abs/sc200919a.html

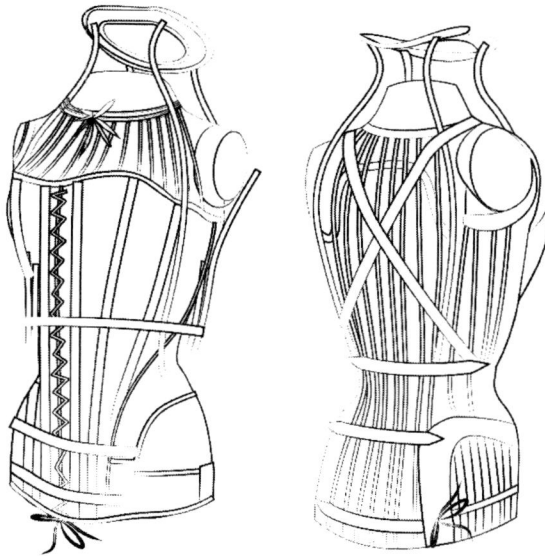

Figure 15. Hessing brace from Germany circa 1888.

In 1835, J. Hossard designed a corset that could be mechanically adjusted to correct spinal curvatures (Figure 16).

Scoliosis Surgery

The first scoliosis surgery was attempted as early as 1839. Jules Guerin was the first to practice a transection (cutting across) of the paraspinal muscles to treat scoliosis. He believed scoliosis developed from an imbalance in the spinal muscles. The results were poor, which is why the method did not become widespread.[55]

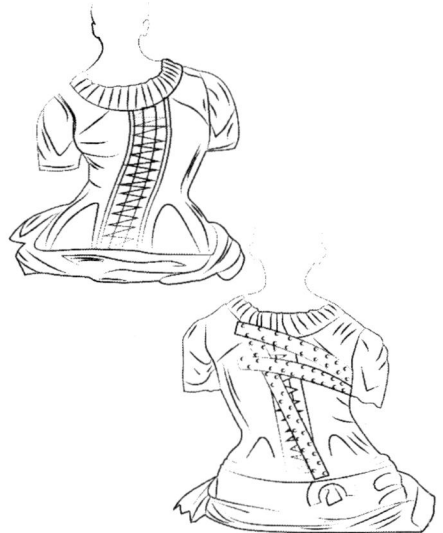

Figure 16. Corrective corset devices by Hossard.

55 Ambrosio L, Tanner E. Biomaterials for spinal surgery. Amsterdam: Elsevier; 2012.

L. Wullstein made an important contribution to the understanding of scoliosis in 1902 with his publication, "Die Skoliose in ihrer Behandlung und Entstehung" ("Scoliosis in its treatment and development"), which documented his clinical and experimental research on scoliosis (Figure 17, 18 & 19).[56]

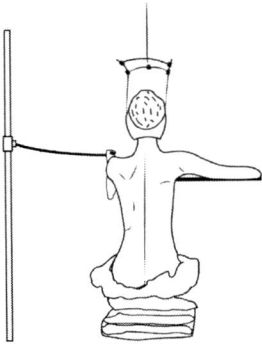

Figure 17. Wullstein scoliosis therapy.

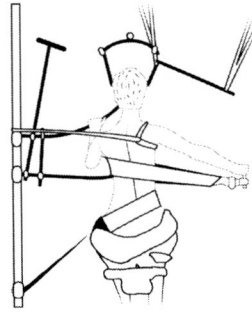

Figure 18. Wullstein scoliosis therapy.

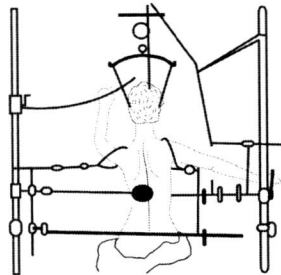

Figure 19. Wullstein scoliosis therapy.

Treatments in the 19th and early 20th centuries included exercises for strengthening the back muscles, as well as casts, braces and combinations of traction, suspension, bracing and postural corrections.

---

56 "Die Skoliose in Ihrer Behandlung und Entstehung nach ..." 2013. 20 Apr. 2016 http://www.worldcat.org/title/skoliose-in-ihrer-behandlung-und-entstehung-nach-klinischen-und-experimentellen-studien/oclc/21218666

Here are illustrations of photographs from 1879-1883, taken by Augusta Zetterling, one of the first female photographers in Sweden.[57] Her subject was a girl with scoliosis. (Figure 20). She is shown wearing an early corrective brace in one of the photographs.

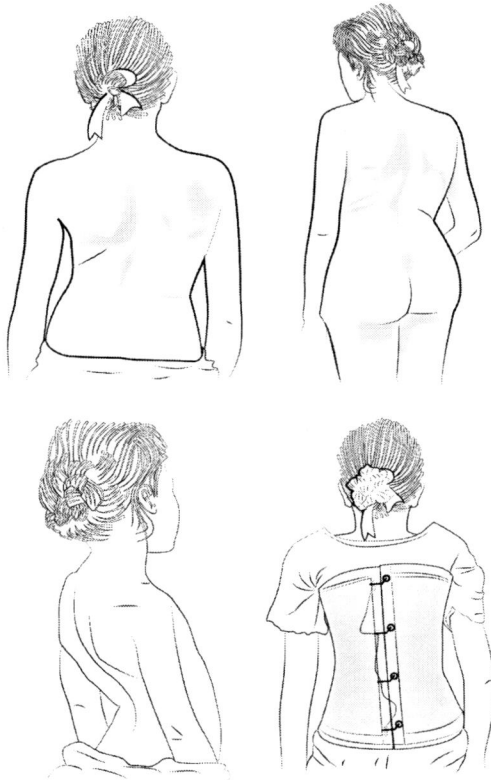

Figure 20. Illustration of photos taken by Augusta Zetterling of a scoliosis patient.

57 "Scoliosis | Wunderkammer." 2012. 20 Apr. 2016 http://wunderkammer.ki.se/images/scoliosis

Chapter 19. Innovations in Adult Scoliosis Bracing

Years ago, one never saw an adult with braces on their teeth, but nowadays it is quite common. Well, nothing is as powerful as an idea whose time has arrived! Yes, adults can now benefit greatly from scoliosis bracing. In this chapter, I will give you a background on scoliosis bracing for adults and provide evidence as to why specific bracing types can be a poor choice for both idiopathic scoliosis in adults and de novo scoliosis. Other bracing types can, in certain situations, be the best option. I will explain why adult bracing for scoliosis MUST be accompanied by specific scoliosis exercises that have been custom designed for that person, that spine, that brace prescription.

Conventional scoliosis braces were not originally developed or designed to treat adults. The origins of the modern scoliosis brace go all the way back to designs from the 16th Century! Over the past 500 years this original concept has seen many modifications, innovations, and entire conceptual breakthroughs. We are fortunate to be able to now apply the advanced stabilization concepts to adult scoliosis patients giving the practitioner an additional powerful tool to help the adult patient whether an ASA or DDS.

How about using a really effective custom-designed brace that has a solid chance of helping adult scoliosis sufferers? Of course, not every case will respond adequately to even the best of brace designs and a small percentage of the braced adults will eventually require surgery, but brace technology has changed significantly in recent years. We have new materials, new approaches, new design methods, new manufacturing methods. The brace of even 10 years ago is radically deficient compared to the best of the braces available today. Unfortunately, almost all orthopedic surgeons and orthotists (Orthotists design and fabricate medical supportive devices and measure and fit patients for them) are still refusing to consider bracing adult scoliosis patients.

There are two groups of patients who can use scoliosis bracing. The first group includes young people who have not reached skeletal maturity. Their braces are meant to be used while the spine is still growing. The second group comprises skeletally mature patients of various ages. This second group includes both de novo (degenerative) adult scoliosis patients as well as adults with adolescent idiopathic scoliosis.

Before we look at modern bracing approaches, let's look back in time to see how this concept of bracing has evolved.

History of Scoliosis Bracing

As described above, the history of the scoliosis back brace begins with Ambrose Paré, who is said to be the physician to first use an orthosis. His brace resembled a metal corset and was made by an armorer in 1575 (Figure 1).[58]

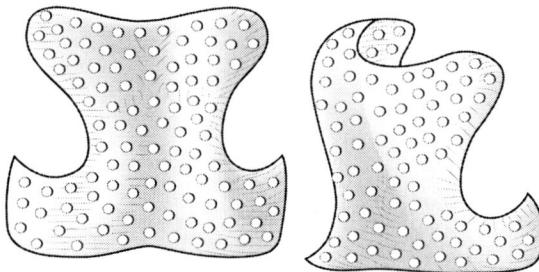

Figure 1. Metal braces by Paré.

Paré decided it was not useful once the person reached skeletal maturity. In 1945, Walter Blount introduced the **Milwaukee Brace** for post-operative immobilization of adolescent scoliosis patients. It was adapted later for non-surgical treatment, becoming one of the most commonly used – but

---

58 Fayssoux, RS. "A History of Bracing for Idiopathic Scoliosis in North America." 2010. 20 Apr. 2016. http://www.ncbi.nlm.nih.gov/pubmed/19462214

not the most effective – scoliosis braces at that time. Today we very rarely see the Milwaukee Brace.

Modern bracing has its foundation in the work of Dr. Jacques Chêneau of Toulouse, France. Chêneau constructed a de-rotation brace out of polyethylene that was presented in 1979 by Professor H. H. Matthiass of Münster as the "**Chêneau Brace**" (Chêneau-Toulouse-Münster, CTM) (Figure 2, C).

During the past 20 years, Dr. Manuel Rigo of Barcelona has furthered the development of the original Chêneau brace by combining his new classification of scoliosis to further customize brace design. His hybrid is called the **Rigo System Chêneau Brace** (RSC Brace) (Figure 2, B).

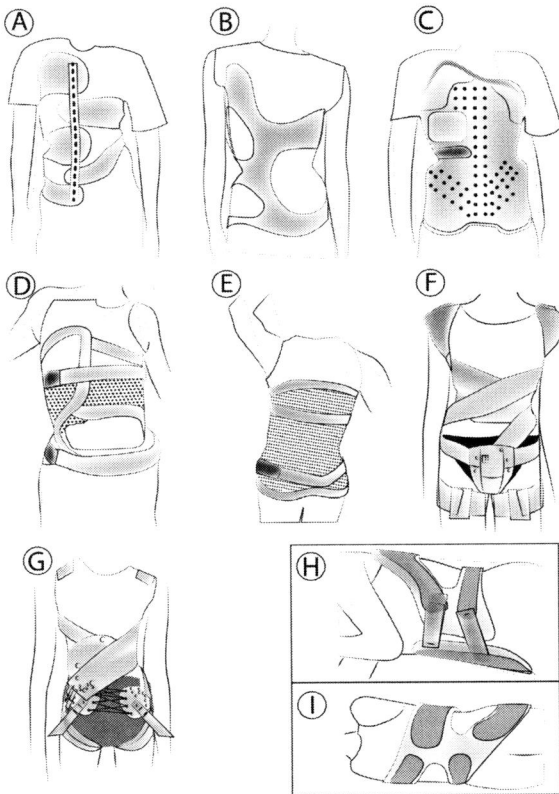

Figure 2. A: Chêneau Light Brace, B: Rigo-System Chêneau (RSC) Brace, C: Chêneau, D&E: Wilmington Brace, F&G: SpineCor Brace, H&I: Providence Brace.

Today, there are a variety of scoliosis braces for children, many of which are named after the city of their original design including the **Boston Brace**, the **Milwaukee Brace**, the **Lyon Brace, and the Wilmington Brace** (Figure 2, D and E). Other braces on the market include the **ART Brace**, the **SPoRT Brace** and the **ScoliBrace**. There are also "part-time" scoliosis braces, designed to be worn only at night, including the **Providence Brace** (Figure 2, H and I) and the Charleston Brace.

The **SpineCor Brace** (Figure 2, F and G), developed at Sainte-Justine Hospital in Montréal by Spine Corp. in 1992, is considered a "dynamic corrective brace." Dynamic corrective braces use soft elastic materials and claim to do more than simply stabilize the progression of scoliosis.[59] The independent research on soft braces (such as SpineCor) reveal that this type of brace is compressive on the curve and therefore of questionable effectiveness on larger curves or on adult patients. Because compressive bands are worn which pull the shoulders downward, they tend to increase the pressure on the curve. Furthermore, the argument that a soft brace overcomes the discomfort issues of a hard brace has proven to be incorrect.[60] Because the soft brace requires the use of a tight girdle to anchor the brace, it too has wearer discomfort issues. In independent scientific literature, the SpineCor brace has been found to have appropriate application only for smaller curves in young, flexible spines.

A new type of brace has been released recently which has application for adult patients, and I use it in cases of progressive adult curves in danger of postural collapse that are not responsive to an exercise-based approach alone. The brace is also used to improve the patient's appearance, especially with painful or unsightly postural side shift. I use the brace in approximately 20-30 percent of the adult cases.

59 "SpineCor Dynamic Corrective Brace." 2013. 22 Apr. 2016 http://www.spinecor. com/ForProfessionals/SpineCorDynamicCorrectiveBrace.aspx

60 Guo, J. "A Prospective Randomized Controlled Study on the Treatment ..." 2014. 26 Apr. 2016. http://link.springer.com/article/10.1007 percent2Fs00586-013-3146-1

Image to the right shows a 2D rendering of a 3D scan of the patient's torso that is used by our brace design software to produce a custom brace.

Each design follows a corrective mirror-image principle applied to each patient's specific imbalance.

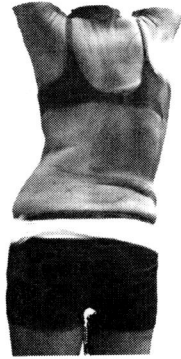

How Does Scientific Research Evaluate Bracing?

There is now very positive research on the effectiveness of scoliosis bracing for adults.

Published in 2016 in the *Archives of Physical Medicine and Rehabilitation,* *Palazzo et. al*[61] studied a group of adult scoliosis over a 15-year period. For 10 years the adults had no treatment and had an average progression of 2 degrees per year or 20 degrees of progression. Researchers then braced the adults for a period of 5 years. During this time, they had a progression of 0.2 degrees per year or 1 degree in 5 years (Figure 3).

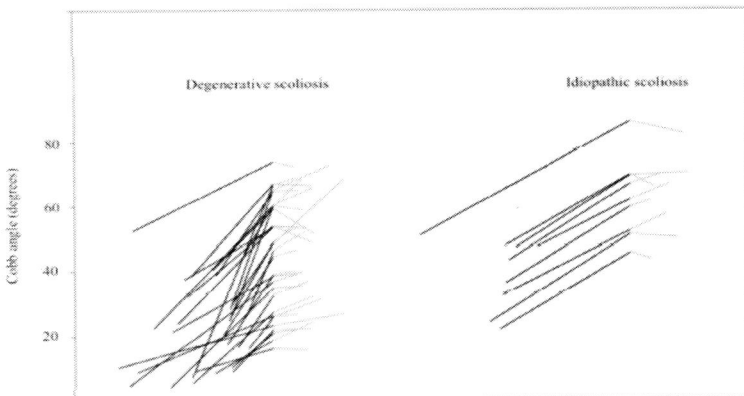

Figure 3. Individual progression of degenerative and idiopathic adult scoliosis before (black) and after bracing (gray line)

---

61 Palazzo, C., et al. "Effects of Bracing in Adult With Scoliosis: A Retrospective Study." *Archives of Physical Medicine and Rehabilitation.* January 2017Volume 98, Issue 1, Pages 187–190

This suggests that bracing may also be a helpful treatment to stop or slow progression in adult scoliosis.

The above figure from Palazzo's article shows each patient's progression of degenerative and idiopathic adult scoliosis before (black line) and after bracing (gray line). Note the downward slope of the grey line showing a decrease in the rate of progression in nearly all cases.

The goals of adult scoliosis bracing differ from the goals of a child's bracing program. In adult patients, our goals are to reduce or eliminate pain, improve the cosmetic appearance of the patient, and prevent the scoliosis from getting worse (preventing postural collapse). Recommended compliance for an adult scoliosis patient is typically to wear the scoliosis brace 4-6 hours per day. If the patient wakes with back pain, wearing the brace during sleep time has proven to be very beneficial.

Many times, I provide a trial period of exercise-based treatment only. If I see the patient would benefit from bracing, I will discuss this with the them. A custom-designed exercise approach is FIRST. The best of the modern braces is the SECOND option. And, surgery should only be considered as a LAST resort!

For over 500 years the traditional scoliosis back brace has been in use. Now three-dimensional imaging technology, combined with modern materials and mirror-image design, has made bracing an effective approach for adults – WHEN NEEDED. It is for these reasons, and based on the evidence, that we use bracing in a selected segment of our patients. Yes, there is a need for bracing at times, but it's much less common among patients using an exercise-based treatment program.

Chapter 20. The History of Scoliosis Surgery

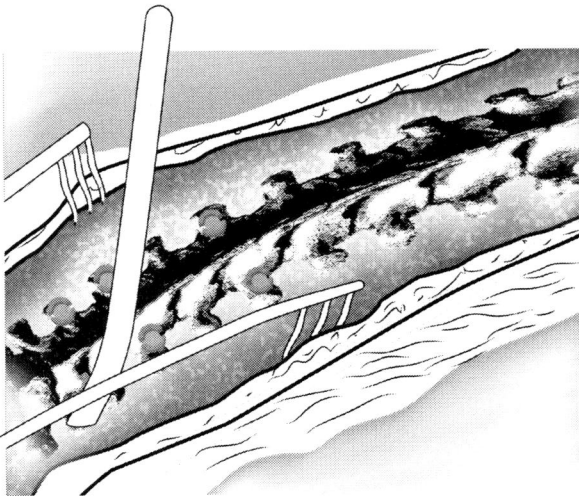

Scoliosis surgery is one of the most complicated orthopedic surgical procedures performed on adults. When conservative treatments like scoliosis exercise programs or bracing are not effective in preventing the progression of the scoliosis, surgery may be prescribed to stop postural collapse. Surgery may even be prescribed sooner if the patient is having uncontrollable severe pain, loss of control of bowels or bladder, or withering of the arms and or legs.

Surgery recommendations for adults vary from a low of 50 degrees all the way up to 80 degrees, depending on the circumstances of the case and the orthopedic specialist consulted. The variation is due to differing philosophies of the orthopedic surgeons specializing in adult scoliosis. While some adults will opt for surgery at the lower threshold to correct cosmetic issues, others will refrain from surgery unless the curve size develops to be very large (over 80 degrees) **AND** there begins to be evidence of heart and/or lung dysfunction.

History of Scoliosis Surgery

The first scoliosis surgeries were on children and were conducted by a French surgeon named Jules Rene Guerin in 1865.[62] This initial surgical attempt to help scoliosis patients involved severing the muscles and tendons of 1,349 patients. This resulted in horrific effects and led to what many consider to be the first recorded instance of medical dispute and one of the most famous orthopedic lawsuits.

Dr. Russell Hibbs performed the first spinal fusion scoliosis surgery at the New York Orthopedic Hospital in 1914. The inventor of spinal fusion surgery; he had been performing the operation on other spinal deformities for three years before applying it to the treatment of a scoliosis caused by tuberculosis.[63][64]

By 1941, spinal fusion operations for adolescents with idiopathic scoliosis were common. The fusions were initially developed to treat tuberculosis, which can affect the spinal bones. Most surgeons (60 percent) used supplemental bone grafts, often from the shin bones. A final curve correction of about 25 percent was achieved. A high complication rate was associated with these early surgeries.

---

62 Ambrosio L, Tanner E. Biomaterials for spinal surgery. Amsterdam: Elsevier; 2012.

63 "The History of Lumbar Spine Stabilization." 2005. 26 Apr. 2016 http://www.burtonreport.com/infspine/SurgStabilSpineHistory.htm

64 "Spinal Fusion: MedlinePlus Medical Encyclopedia." 2006. 26 Apr. 2016 https://www.nlm.nih.gov/medlineplus/ency/article/002968.htm

Twenty years later, Paul Harrington introduced the first use of implanted steel rods to straighten scoliosis surgically. These hooks and rods are known as a spinal instrumentation system. Harrington's original concept was to use spinal instrumentation without fusion.[65]

Due to poor results with just rods, his protocol changed to spinal fusion in conjunction with the Harrington rods. The Harrington Rod procedure was developed in the 1950s. A single inflexible steel rod secured the straightened spine, and bone was grafted from the patient's hip and placed into the verte-bral spaces to stimulate a fusion. This surgery was performed through the back and led to loss of all flexibility in the full length of the fusion. The sur-gery lasted between eight and 12 hours, and recovery was slow and difficult.

The patient would be confined to bed for three to six months in a full body cast from the neck to below the hips and another six months in a hard plas-tic jacket similar to today's Wilmington Brace.

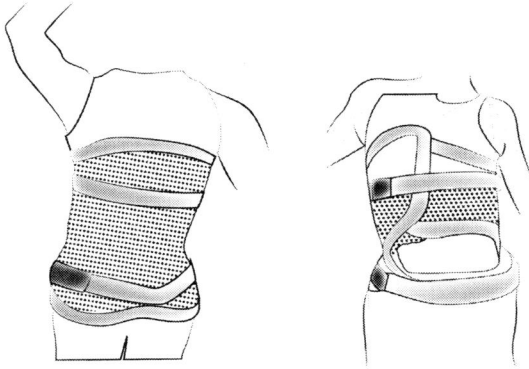

Wilmington Brace

By the mid-70s, the Harrington method often was performed using two rods to correct the upper and lower curves.

---

65 National Scoliosis Foundation. "Instrumentation Systems For Scoliosis Sur-gery". National Scoliosis Foundation. Retrieved February 11, 2010.

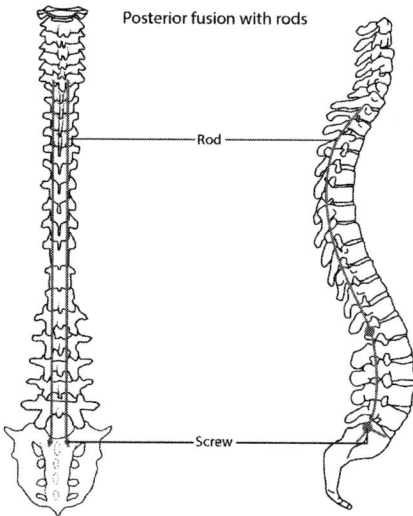

Posterior fusion with rods

Rod

Screw

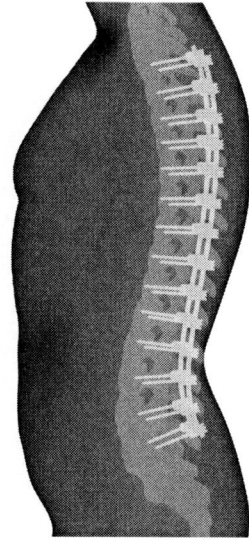

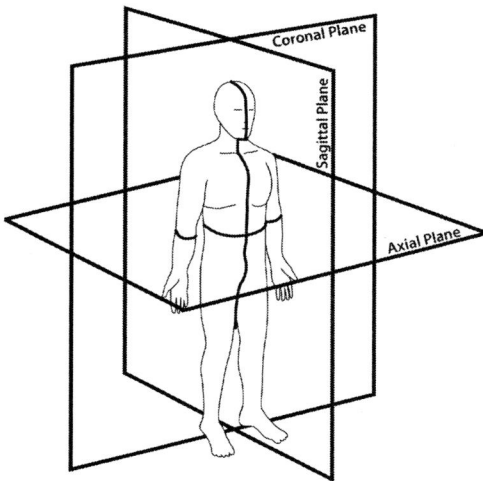

Coronal Plane

Sagittal Plane

Axial Plane

Dr. Yves Cotrel and Dr. Jean Dubousset of France developed the pedicle screw system known as Cotrel-Dubousset (CD) instrumentation. It was the first system that allowed for de-rotation of the spinal bones which corrected scoliosis in the sagittal (front to back) plane in addition to the coronal/lateral (side to side). Although correction rates achieved by posterior pedicle-screw are good overall, the rate of post-scoliosis surgery complications is very high.[66]

One study found that 68 percent of patients experienced minor or major severe complications. Another study determined that there is no significant

66 "Lumbar Fusion | University of Maryland Medical Center." 26 Apr. 2016 http://umm.edu/programs/spine/health/guides/lumbar-fusion

improvement to surgical outcomes by using the CD system over Harrington rods, while the newer CD system is significantly more expensive.[67]

While there is obviously a place for surgery in the treatment of scoliosis, exercise-based programs can be a viable alternative to surgery in many cases.

---

67 Modi, HN. "Scoliosis and Spinal Disorders | Pre-publication history ..." 2009. 26 Apr. 2016. http://www.scoliosisjournal.com/content/4/1/11/prepub

> *"The wisest mind has something yet to learn."*
>
> – **George Santayana**

Chapter 21. Lung Function and Scoliosis

Because the thoracic spine is part of the rib cage, which stores vital organs such as the heart and lungs, significant scoliosis in the thoracic spine can affect heart and lung function. Studies have shown a significant correlation between lung and heart function and the degree of scoliosis in patients with very large thoracic-dominant curves. Here we are talking about scoliosis greater than 70-80 degrees.

"Twenty-two (22 percent) of 98 patients complained of shortness of breath during everyday activities compared with eight (15 percent) of 53 controls. An increased risk of shortness of breath was also associated with the combination of a Cobb angle greater than 80 degrees and a thoracic apex (adjusted odds ratio, 9.75; 95 percent CI, 1.15-82.98). Sixty-six (61 percent) of 109 patients reported chronic back pain compared with 22 (35 percent) of 62 controls (P =.003). However, of those with pain, 48 (68 percent) of 71 patients and 12 (71 percent) of 17 controls reported only little or moderate back pain."[68]

Another study which confirms these findings concludes, "Pulmonary and cardiac function was significantly correlated with the degree of scoliosis in patients with thoracic-dominant scoliosis." [69]

---

68 Weinstein, SL. "Health and Function of Patients with Untreated ... - NCBI." 2003. 26 Apr. 2016. http://www.ncbi.nlm.nih.gov/pubmed/12578488

69 Huh, S. "Cardiopulmonary Function and Scoliosis Severity in ... – NCBI." 2015. 26 Apr. 2016. http://www.ncbi.nlm.nih.gov/pmc/articles/PMC4510355/

In another study, twenty-four patients who had not received scoliosis sur-gery were examined in 1968 and then re-examined 20 years later to deter-mine if any changes in lung function had occurred. **Researchers found that decline in lung function over the 20 years was the same as the predicted decline due to aging.** Patients' lung function measurement from 1968 was the strongest predictor of developing respiratory failure, followed by their curve size. Respiratory failure occurred only in patients who had a lung function measurement below 45 percent in 1968 and whose curves were greater than 110 degrees. Thus, respiratory failure develops in adults with scoliosis who have large curves and low lung function when normal aging further reduces lung function. [70]

Does scoliosis surgery fix this type of lung problem? Unfortunately, the an-swer is usually "No."

In *Scoliosis and the Human Spine*, Dr. Martha Hawes, Ph.D., the author, talks candidly about the impact of surgery on lung dysfunction:

"If pulmonary dysfunction were a consequence of spinal curvature per se, then improving the magnitude of curvature would be predicted to result in a corresponding improvement in pulmonary function. However, instead [the pulmonary dysfunction] is due to a secondary loss of skeletal mobility. Fur-ther reductions in spinal and skeletal mobility beyond those associated with the spinal deformity being treated is one of the complications of spinal fusion surgery. Therefore, it is not surprising that surgically-induced improvement in Cobb Angle is not correlated with a matching increases in respiratory function and that pulmonary function may in fact decline after surgery (Bjure, 1969; Goldberg, 2002; Katz and Kumar, 1983; Kinnear, 1992; Lenke, 1995; Lenke, 2002; Sakic, 1992; Upadhyay, 1994)."

"In summary, after recovery from a significant decline in respiratory function due to the surgery per se there ultimately may be a slight improvement in pul-monary function, or there may be a decrease, or there may be no change at all

70 Pehrsson,K, Bake,B, Larsson, S, Nachemson, A. "Lung function in adult idio-pathic scoliosis: a 20 year follow up." —NCBI. 1991. https://www.ncbi.nlm.nih.gov/pmc/articles/PMC463231/

(Kishan, 2007; Vedantam, 2000; Koumbourlis, 2006; McCool and Rochester, 2000; Newton and Wenger, 2001; Seaton, 2000). *Physicians are advised to let their patients know that improved pulmonary function, let alone a significant improvement, is not a reasonable expectation of spine surgery* (Bowen, 1995)."

"*Impact of spine surgery on signs & symptoms of spinal deformity," again by Hawes, states: "For most patients, there is little or no improvement in pulmonary function." Hawes also mentions that, "Since 1995, only 9 of 93 papers on "scoliosis surgery" have included spirometry to measure pulmonary function as part of the outcome. With one exception, these recent reports confirm previous studies indicating that, **irrespective of severity of curvature or surgical approach, improved curvature magnitude does not result in significantly improved *VC, **TLC, or exercise capacity."* [71]

Let's connect the dots here... What does decreased lung function due to very large scoliosis mean with regard to lifespan? How does decreased lung function affect the lifespan of patients with very large curves?

Let's look at the Framingham Heart Study data. Physicians reviewing the data from the study concluded that **"your lungs are the number one predictor of death."** This is not a scoliosis study; however, the conclusions are very valuable for understanding the importance of proper lung function.

The Framingham Heart Study is a medical study that started in 1948 and has followed a population of thousands for six decades. The original researchers recruited over 5,200 men and women from Framingham, Mass. At that time, study participants were free of any cardiovascular disease.

In 1971, the study enrolled adult children of original participants and their spouses, and in 1994 additional subjects were enrolled in order to create a more diverse study population. In 2002, a third generation – the grandchildren of the original participants – started enrolling.

The Framingham Study is one of the oldest, largest and most prestigious ongoing medical studies in the world. One of the focuses of their study was the

---

71 *Vital Capacity, **Total Lung Capacity

long-term predictive effects of vital capacity and forced exhalation volume (lung function) as a primary marker for lifespan.

Here's what the Framingham doctors wrote:

"Pulmonary function measurement (a measure of lung function) appears to be an indicator of general health and vigor and literally a measure of living capacity. . . Long before a person becomes terminally ill, vital capacity can predict lifespan. The Framingham examinations' predictive powers were as accurate over the 30-year period as were more recent exams." [72]

In other words, lung capacity predicted lifespan as accurately as any other exams.

72 Mahmood, SS. "The Framingham Heart Study and the Epidemiology ... – NCBI." 2014. 25 Apr. 2016. http://www.ncbi.nlm.nih.gov/pmc/articles/PMC4159698/

Chapter 22. A Disturbing Report on Scoliosis Surgery

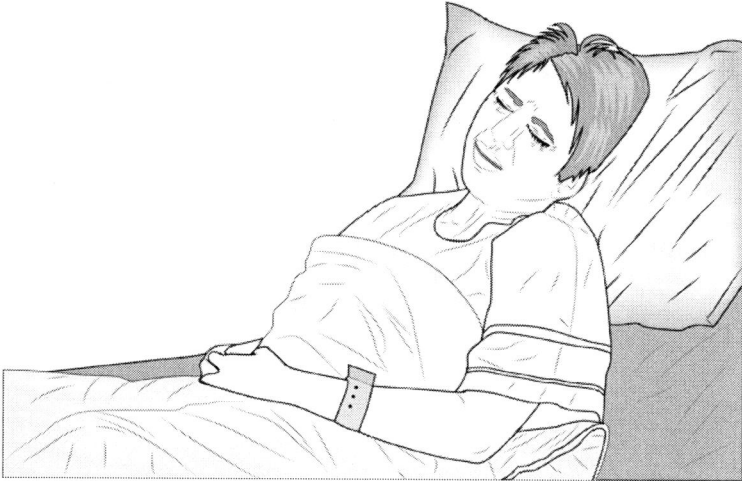

Yes, there is a time when surgery is absolutely the right thing to do in scoliosis treatment. When severe adolescent idiopathic scoliosis in the adult or de novo scoliosis progresses to a point at which there is strong pain, severe nerve damage effecting the internal organs or limb strength, or lung and heart function are compromised, surgery can become a necessary intervention. Spinal fusion surgery on a large scoliosis is a very complex and invasive medically necessary surgical procedure that can result in strong postoperative pain. A 2013 study detailed the experiences of patients (ages 8-25) who underwent corrective spinal surgery between 2004-2007, and the results were an unsettlingly consistent tale of extreme pain, debilitating nausea and an overwhelming sense of helplessness.[73] If it is this bad for a young person, you can only imagine how hard it can be on a mature adult.

A 2012 study[74] detailed the risks associated with scoliosis surgery in adults. This was a large French multicenter study which looked at 306 adults ages ranging from 50-83 with curves around 50 degrees. They found the overall complication rate was 39 percent, and 26 percent of the patients were operated on again for mechanical or neurological complications. There is a 44 percent risk of a new operation in the 6-year-period after the primary procedure.

Isaacs, Robert E. MD; Hyde, Jonathan MD; Goodrich, J. et al determined that the rate of major complications for surgical fusion treatment of adult degenerative scoliosis was 12.1 percent. This statistic is similar to that reported from other studies of surgery for degenerative deformity.[75]

Dr. S. Kotwal , confirms that the incidence of surgical complications for the adult scoliosis patient are substantial and the surgeon and patient must discuss this fully when considering a surgical option.

Here is a direct quote from another study on the complications associated with adult degenerative scoliosis:

"Adult degenerative scoliosis surgery is a complex undertaking. The surgeries are large and intricate. The patient population is typically sick and debilitated. Because of these factors, complications frequently arise."[76]

---

73 Rullander, AC. "Young People's Experiences with Scoliosis Surgery: a Survey ..." 2013. 26 Apr. 2016. http://www.ncbi.nlm.nih.gov/pubmed/24247313

74 Charosky S, Guigui P, Blamoutier A, Roussouly P, Chopin D. Complications and risk factors of primary adult scoliosis surgery: a multicenter study of 306 patients. Spine (Phila Pa 1976). 2012;37(8):693–700

75 Isaacs, RE, Hyde, J., Goodrich, J.A; Rodgers, WB, Phillips, F. "A Prospective, Nonrandomized, Multicenter Evaluation of Extreme Lateral Interbody Fusion for the Treatment of Adult Degenerative Scoliosis: Perioperative Outcomes and Complications." Spine: Dec., 2010 35(26S). S322-S330. https://journals.lww.com/spine-journal/Abstract/2010/12151/A_Prospective,_Nonrandomized,_Multicenter.8.aspx

76 Shridharani, S.,Munroe, B., Hood, K. "Complications in adult degenerative scoliosis surgery." *Seminars in Spine Surgery. 29(2). June 2017. 118-122.*

When surgical treatment is selected for adult degenerative scoliosis, it is vital to consider the risks. Older patients usually have other medical conditions so the incidence of complications occurring around the time of the surgery, such as cardiopulmonary insufficiency, deep vein thrombosis and infection, are quite high. The most common issue for the older scoliosis patient considering surgery is osteoporosis. Osteoporosis can weaken the strength of the fusion, causing loss of correction and pseudarthrosis (failure of the fusion). [77]

A study on adolescent scoliosis surgery found, on average, most postoperative pain was described as severe and lasting for roughly five days. Of those adolescents, 60 percent also reported "persistent pain or recent onset pain 5-12 months after surgery." Patients from the study detailed experiences of mismanagement and unbearable pain while getting in and out of bed, standing and during chest tube removal.

"I felt like I was hung up on meat hooks."

"Sometimes it feels like a knife is cutting into my back."

As one can imagine, pain management is an essential part of recovery and can involve epidural, intravenous, and also spinal analgesics. However, these medications come with their own sets of side effects: nausea, constipation, pruritus (itching), urinary retention, sedation, respiratory depression, and decreased blood pressure.

Nausea was another common complaint. The nausea persisted for an average of three days, though some patients experienced it for the duration of their hospital stay or even after they left. Parents reported drug treatment as ineffective and that the nausea only subsided when opioid medication doses were decreased. Some patients reported not eating while in the hospital because of nausea, and some even felt the nausea was worse than the pain.

---

77 Cho, K, Kim,Y,Shin, S., Suk, S. "Surgical Treatment of Adult Degenerative Scoliosis." *Asian Spine Journal.* 2014 Jun; 8(3): 371–381. https://www.ncbi.nlm.nih.gov/pmc/articles/PMC4068860/

The most heart-breaking detail of this study were the parents' feelings of helplessness as their children were suffering. Parents and patients described inadequacies of nursing staff, failure of pain control equipment, anxiety, nightmares, and too much time spent waiting for assistance. The authors indicate that "symptoms of post-traumatic stress were vividly described in narrative interviews with some of the adolescents."

"She had fear in her eyes. We have never seen that expression before. She cannot express herself you know! I can't remember whether she screamed or moaned or if she stared at us with pure fear trying to say – help me!"

"Everything was OK until the catheter with analgesics stopped functioning. After that there were several difficult days with severe pain. My daughter has had nightmares about pain since then."

"It was terrible to see my daughter having so much pain and not being able to help her."[78]

What's shocking, though, is that parents and patients alike rated their over-all hospital stay as satisfactory. Researchers suggested such a discrepancy may exist because satisfaction was based on other factors, including that they expected such an experience.

Since this study, pain management techniques have been modified to include "patient-controlled epidural analgesia." However, the authors are quick to add that the most painful instances were when the epidural catheters failed and when patients were switched from the catheters to oral medications.

---

78 Rullander, Anna-Clara et al. "Young People's Experiences with Scoliosis Surgery: a Survey of Pain, Nausea, and Global Satisfaction." *Orthopaedic Nursing* 32.6 (2013): 327-333. Print.

> *From Physician-Patient Alliance for Health & Safety (PPAHS.ORG):*
>
> *"Patient Controlled Analgesia (PCA) pumps were developed to address the problem of under medication. They are used to permit the patient to self-administer small doses of narcotics (usually Morphine, Dilaudid, Demerol, or Fentanyl) into the blood or spinal fluid at frequent intervals. PCA pumps are commonly used after surgery to provide a more effective method of pain control than periodic injections of narcotics."[79]*

Another 2013 study on postoperative pain from spinal fusion surgery assessed pain scores, use of opioids, and the recovery process. It stated:

"The standard of care for pain management for spine surgery in children consists of continuous infusion of intravenous (IV) morphine supplemented with patient-controlled analgesia (PCA). However, to achieve satisfactory pain control with this method, high doses of opioids must be administered. Unfortunately, use of opioids is associated with serious adverse effects, including nausea, vomiting, pruritus, sedation, and respiratory depression, which often delay patient recovery."[80]

Surgery for all but the largest curve (0.1 percent of scoliosis cases) should be called what it really is: "elective spinal fusion surgery." ELECTIVE, not NECESSARY. Patients need to be fully informed that surgery is a treatment choice and is rarely a necessity. A custom-designed exercise program and over-corrective bracing when appropriate are a choice in the vast majority of scoliosis cases in adults.

Let's look at two excerpts from two different *Spine* articles about the discouraging outcome of some spinal implant removals:

---

79 "Patient Controlled Analgesia (PCA) Pumps: The Basics." 2015. 25 Apr. 2016 http://www.ppahs.org/2012/05/patient-controlled-analgesia-pca-pumps-the-basics/

80 Reynolds, RA. "Postoperative Pain Management after Spinal Fusion Surgery ..." 2013. 26 Apr. 2016. http://www.ncbi.nlm.nih.gov/pubmed/24436846

"Despite bony fusion, loss of correction between 10 degrees and 26 degrees was observed in three patients after instrumentation removal."[81]

"Spinal implant removal after long posterior fusion in adults may lead to spinal collapse and further surgery. Removal of instrumentation should be avoided or should involve partial removal of the prominent implant." [82]

That's hard to read, isn't it?

81 Hahn, Frederik, Reinhard Zbinden, and Kan Min. "Late Implant Infections Caused by Propionibacterium Acnes in Scoliosis Surgery." *European Spine Journal* 14.8 (2005): 783-788. Print.

82 Deckey, Jeffrey E, and David S Bradford. "Loss of Sagittal Plane Correction after Removal of Spinal Implants." *Spine* 25.19 (2000): 2453-2460. Print.

> "We live in a world of constant juxtaposition between joy that's possible and pain that's all too common. We hope for love and success and abundance, but we never quite forget that there is always lurking the possibility of disaster."
>
> – Marianne Williamson

Chapter 23. Can Spinal Rods, Hooks and Surgical Screws Break?

The Long Term Effects of Adolescent Scoliosis Surgery on Patients Now Entering Middle Age

Steel alloy and even titanium rods can bend, break loose from their wires, or worse, break completely in two, necessitating further surgical intervention and removal of the rods.[83] Once the rod is removed, corrosion is found on two out of every three patients.[84]

Recent studies are showing concern about the possible toxic effect on the body of having a large metallic implant for decades. One study suggests that the presence of metallic particles from titanium-alloy pedicle screw hardware may be the cause of late-onset inflammatory response and late operative-site pain.[85]

---

83 "Scoliosis Surgery: Things to Consider-OrthoInfo – AAOS." 2011. 25 Apr. 2016 http://orthoinfo.aaos.org/topic.cfm?topic=A00641

84 Akazawa, Tsutomu et al. "Corrosion of Spinal Implants Retrieved from Patients with Scoliosis." *Journal of Orthopaedic Science* 10.2 (2005): 200-205. Print.

85 Kim, HD. "Electron Microprobe Analysis and Tissue Reaction ... – NCBI." 2007. 26 Apr. 2016. http://www.ncbi.nlm.nih.gov/pmc/articles/PMC2857498/

Though, complication due to metal hypersensitivity is rare, some studies suggest that cases involving implant-related metal sensitivity are underreported because they are difficult to diagnosis.[86][87][88][89]

Prospective studies have shown a higher incidence of metal hypersensitivity in patients with implant failure.[90] Researchers suggest that metal hypersensitivity after spinal fusion should be suspected in patients with postoperative back pain and that an elaborate case history would lead to a correct diagnosis.[91]

"The brief answer to our initial question is yes, patients can be allergic to hardware if they have a pre-existing allergy to the materials that make up the hardware (titanium, stainless steel, etc.). Your surgical team will do a thorough investigation of your existing allergies prior to your procedure to avoid any potential allergic reactions after surgery. However, certain allergies can develop over time. So, a person who has already had spinal hardware put in place can potentially develop an allergy to it years down the line.

An allergic reaction can crop up in the form of headaches, pain in the back and extremities, fever, and other symptoms. If you notice any severe symptoms

86 Thyssen, Jacob Pontoppidan et al. "The Association Between Metal Allergy, Total Hip Arthroplasty, and Revision: A Case-Control Study." *Acta Orthopaedica* 80.6 (2009): 646-652. Print.

87 Shang, X. "Metal Hypersensitivity in Patient with Posterior Lumbar Spine ..." 2014. 25 Apr. 2016. http://bmcmusculoskeletdisord.biomedcentral.com/articles/10.1186/1471-2474-15-314

88 Jokar, M. "Epidemiology of Vasculitides in Khorasan Province, Iran." 2015. 26 Apr. 2016. http://www.ncbi.nlm.nih.gov/pmc/articles/PMC4487463/

89 Thyssen, Jacob Pontoppidan et al. "The Association Between Metal Allergy, Total Hip Arthroplasty, and Revision: A Case-Control Study." *Acta Orthopaedica* 80.6 (2009): 646-652. Print.

90 Frigerio, E. "Metal Sensitivity in Patients with Orthopaedic Implants: a ..." 2011. 26 Apr. 2016. http://www.ncbi.nlm.nih.gov/pubmed/21480913

91 Shang, Xianping et al. "Metal Hypersensitivity in Patient with Posterior Lumbar Spine Fusion: a Case Report and its Literature Review." *BMC Musculoskeletal Disorders* 15.1 (2014): 314. Print.

after your spine surgery, be sure to contact your surgeon. It may be necessary to remove the spinal hardware to avoid any further complications." [92]

Below, is an illustration of X-rays of an individual with broken spinal rods. This adult had spinal fusion as a teen, but now needs a revision surgery to deal with the broken rod.

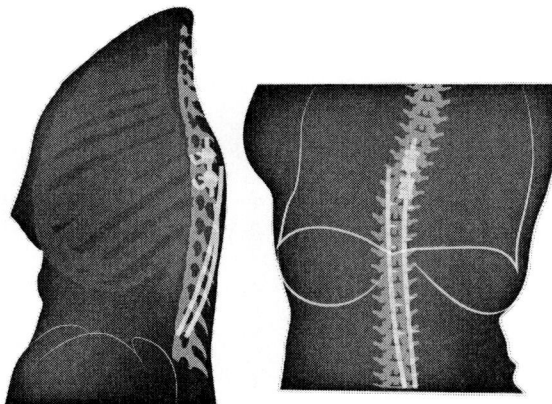

The above illustration of X-rays depicts steel alloy rods that bent and broke while still inside the patient's body. Many surgeons will refuse to operate on this condition, leaving the patient with few options to alleviate their pain and suffering.[93]

Rod removal is usually considered when there is local pain at the site of a broken rod or from a prominent hook. Often, however, only part of a rod or one or more prominent hooks can be removed to relieve symptoms. The spinal fusions are often extremely solid, and the new bone formation encases the rods and the hooks; therefore, removal of the entire rod may not be possible, and one or more hooks may be left behind. The wound then needs two to three weeks to heal unless there is additional bone grafting needed.

92 "Can You Be Allergic to Spine Hardware? | Dr. Stefano ..." 2014. 25 Apr. 2016 http://sinicropispine.com/can-allergic-spine-hardware/

93 "Scoliosis Surgery: Things to Consider-OrthoInfo – AAOS." 2011. 25 Apr. 2016 http://orthoinfo.aaos.org/topic.cfm?topic=A00641

Some curvatures continue to progress after spinal fusion due to broken rods or other instrument failure. In a paper about the role of Harrington instrumentation and posterior spine fusion in AIS patients, researcher T.S. Renshaw said that, *"One would expect that if the patient lives long enough, rod breakage will be a virtual certainty."* [94]

Furthermore, discomfort may occur when any pressure is placed against the back; this is especially problematic with newer bulky instrumentation implanted in thin patients, noted researcher H.R. Weiss in his 2008 study about AIS and surgery. [95]

Even with a solid fusion, a small percentage of Harrington rods subsequently fracture, due to micro-movement in daily activities. When rods break within two years of operation, it usually indicates fusion failure (pseudarthrosis) and it will need to be surgically repaired by more bone grafting and possible modification of the rods. [96]

Here are what those on online forums say when discussing complications, pain and discomfort from malfunctioning Harrington rods:

"My dad has had metal rods in his back since 1995. They are horrible. He is in so much more pain than before and now every doctor says there is nothing they can do for him b/c the rods can never come out. I am trying to get him into the mayo clinic but so far haven't had any luck. He lives in constant pain."

To read more, go to: Orthopedics Forum – Broken Harrington Rod
http://ehealthforum.com/health/topic10952.html#ixzz1x8lgiY42

"Hello, I too had scoliosis surgery when I was like 12 or 13. I am now 31. I had/ have been having a lot of back pain. Last summer I went back to the dr. that

---

94 Renshaw, T. S. "The Role of Harrington Instrumentation and Posterior Spine Fusion in the Management of Adolescent Idiopathic Scoliosis." *The Orthopedic Clinics of North America* 19.2 (1988): 257-267. Print.

95 Weiss, HR. "Adolescent Idiopathic Scoliosis – to Operate or Not? A ... – NCBI." 2008. 26 Apr. 2016. http://www.ncbi.nlm.nih.gov/pmc/articles/PMC2572584/

96 "Scoliosis Research Society." 2015. 25 Apr. 2016 https://www.srs.org/chinese_sim/patient_and_family/the_aging_spine/pseudarthrosis.htm

did the surgery. That is when I found out that my rod is broken. I don't know when it happened. I just know I have constant pain in my shoulder blade on up. So, unfortunately, yes, the rod can break. But, I do not know the solution."

To read more, go to: National Scoliosis Foundation Forums http://www.scoliosis.org/forum/archive/index.php/t-210.html

"My daughter had her titanium Harrington rods removed on May 24th. She was two years post injury, and had constant, deep pain in her lower back. She was also constantly nauseated, making it difficult to eat."

To read more, go to: CareCure Forums – Removal of Harrington Rods http://sci.rutgers.edu/forum/showthread.php?3361-Removal-of-Harrington-Rods

"I was told the best they could do as a last resort would be to cut off pieces at each end of the break. To keep the broken halves from banging into each other. The rods were grafted/fused to my back using pieces of my hip. I was told to remove them would be extremely difficult and there was a good chance I'd be worse off afterward."

To read more, go to: Spina Bifida Connection Support Forum-Broken Harrington Rod Pics http://spinabifidaconnection.com/archive/index.php/t-767.html

> *"We are built to conquer environment, solve problems, achieve*
> *goals, and we find no real satisfaction or happiness in life without*
> *obstacles to conquer and goals to achieve."*
>
> **– Maxwell Maltz**

Chapter 24. Can Patients View Scoliosis Surgery as 'Failed'?

If scoliosis surgery is so problematic, why is it that the majority of patients say they are pleased with the process?

A 2008 research review of of existing studies on the complications associated with scoliosis surgery discussed the possible influence of a psychological effect called "cognitive dissonance" in scoliosis surgery outcomes. Cognitive dissonance theory tells us that people have an internal psychological need to hold all their attitudes and beliefs in harmony and will not tolerate disharmony, or dissonance. Any psychological "discomfort" that comes from feeling like one has made a bad decision leads to an alteration of their attitudes, beliefs or behaviors to reduce the discomfort/anxiety and restore comfort/harmony. [97]

The authors of the study postulated that this type of discomfort may be occurring in patients who have a high rate of complications with scoliosis surgery, but still report they are happy with their decision. It also suggests that the rate of complications may be higher than reported.

"Instead of achieving long-term evidence for surgical treatment on a higher level and addressing the problems after surgery to attempt to improve patient's safety, the surgical community is presenting large numbers of papers describ-

---

97 Weiss, Hans-Rudolf, and Deborah Goodall. "Rate of Complications in Scoliosis Surgery–a Systematic Review of the Pub Med Literature." *Scoliosis* 3.1 (2008): 1. 22 Apr. 2016.

ing HRQL (Health Related Quality of Life Questionnaires) after surgery and related research [223-241]. The problem with such studies however, is that they lack validity as they do not investigate the actual signs of scoliosis or the symptoms of the patient post-surgery [242]."

The studies containing psychological questionnaires may be compromised by the dissonance effect [242-246]. Unable to face an inconsistency, such as being dissatisfied with a surgical procedure, a person will often change their attitude or action. Surgery is impossible to reverse, but subjective beliefs and public attitude can be altered more easily. In terms of research, this is important because a patient not satisfied with scoliosis surgery may not admit it. [242]"[98]

The authors of the study also give examples of the dissonance effect as reflected in scoliosis literature: "Radiographic and physical measures of deformity do not correlate well with patients' and parents' perceptions of appearance. Patients and parents do not strongly agree on the cosmetic outcome of AIS surgery." (Figure 1)

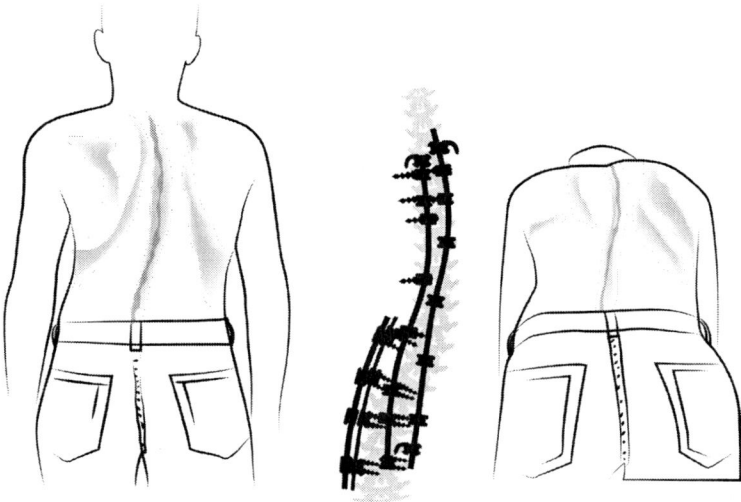

Figure 1. Patient's surgical outcome used as example in the study.

---

98 Ibid.

*"Not the best clinical result with patient satisfaction. This patient was sat-isfied although two operations have been necessary, and the rib-hump and decompensation are still visible. **This satisfaction may be the result of the dissonance effect** [242]."* [99]

*"Today, from the patient's perspective, **health care professionals have more open questions than answers when approaching the subject of spinal sur-gery in patients with scoliosis**. For example; What are the long-term effects in the elderly; how long does the cosmetic effect of an operation last; is there a prospective controlled study clearly showing that scoliosis surgery really pre-vents progression in the long term; does the untreated patient really feel more impaired when progressing 10 degrees more in 20 years?"* [100]

Another more recent study by the same authors (Weiss et al., 2013) yet again addressed the lack of regard for cognitive dissonance in scoliosis literature. They suggest that spinal fusion for adolescent idiopathic scoliosis should only be considered when it is the rare curve that has progressed to a very severe degree or in patients with substantial psychological trauma due sco-liosis deformity. "However, this is rarely the case in a population treated conservatively according to the latest standards," Weiss said.

Most importantly, medical policy stresses the need for informed consent to document patient awareness and a surgeon's liability in patients requir-ing surgery. Patients need to be aware of the high percentage of long-term complications of fusion surgery and the extent of long-term complications [15,16,17]. [101] (Hawes,2006; Weiss et al., 2008; Mueller, 2012)

"The stress the patient experiences due to the deformity must be docu-mented," said Weiss. He also noted:

---

99 Ibid.

100 Ibid.

101 Weiss HR, Moramarco M, Moramarco K. "Risks and long-term complications of adolescent idiopathic scoliosis surgery versus non-surgical and natural history outcomes." *Hard Tissue* 2013 Apr 30;2(3):27.

"It is highly recommended that patients complete the preoperative patient awareness documentation regarding possible complications, <u>sometimes presenting more than 20 years post-operatively</u> [15,16,17]. This documentation, in conjunction with the deformity-related stress level questionnaire, should be read carefully for full disclosure of long-term effects."[102] (2008)

The authors conclude, "A medical indication for AIS spinal fusion surgery does not exist, except in extreme cases. The rate of complications of spinal fusion surgery appears to increase with time. The risk/reward relationship of spinal fusion surgery is unfavourable for the AIS patient, except in rare cases. There is no evidence that spinal fusion surgery improves quality of life for AIS patients versus natural history. The risks and long-term costs, in terms of pain and suffering, after spinal fusion surgery exceeds what is reasonable for AIS patients, putting the common practice of surgery in question, except in extreme cases."[103]

---

102 Ibid.

103 Ibid.

Chapter 25. Orthopedists and the Potential for Conflict of Interest

Why Do Orthopedists Discourage Alternative Scoliosis Treatments Even When Patients Show Improvement from Them?

The medical approach to adult scoliosis treatment is to watch and wait, prescribe over the counter pain meds and general PT, and then in severe cases operate. During the "wait and see" period, orthopedists generally do not advise patients about alternative treatment options, and some even laugh or scoff at the suggestion. Patients are made to feel absurd if they want to pursue proactive or preventative treatments during this pre-surgery period and instead are advised to just sit idly while their curves progress until surgery become "necessary."

Some patients choose to research treatment and try alternative treatments anyway, but upon re-evaluation by their doctor they are told they are wasting their time! Some patients are belittled, made to feel foolish, and some are even harassed by their orthopedist.

If there are fewer risks with alternative treatments, if these approaches are received while patients are in the "watch and wait" period, and if these treatments show improvement to the patient's pain, posture, and even reduce the scoliosis, then why is the medical community so against them?

Do Orthopedists Fail to Suggest Early-Intervention Exercise Programs or Other Alternative Scoliosis Treatments Because of a Conflict of Interest?

If you have surgery and it fails, exercise-based care programs will only be able to target the non-operated areas of the spine. Hooks, screws and stabilizing devices in your spine will impede exercise-based programs targeting those areas. If you have an exercise-based program that, in the rare case, is not successful, the surgeon will always be waiting for you. It is the rare adult case that could not stand to wait a year or so to see what kind of benefit conservative care could offer. And... the improved core strength and mobility you gain from the specialized exercises would probably actually help the surgeon achieve a higher degree of correction and help you to have a faster more complete recovery.

In Martha C. Hawes' book *Scoliosis and the Human Spine (2010), the University of Arizona professor and research scientist outlines what appears to be a conflict of interest in the medical community. The conflict centers upon the general lack of regard for exercise-based programs of scoliosis care and correction. Let's take a closer look.*

Do Nothing (Watch and Wait)

Dr. Hawes, Ph.D., who has ASA (Adolescent Scoliosis in an Adult) herself, said:

"We have the wherewithal to diagnose spinal deformity at a Cobb magnitude of ten degrees or less, before it progresses to a serious problem that may cause pain, deformity, psychological dysfunction, and pulmonary problems throughout the patient's lifetime. But instead of making an effort to diagnose the underlying condition and take steps to stabilize or reverse the curvature at this relatively benign state (and despite longstanding basic and clinical research consistent with the hypothesis that this is entirely feasible), patients and parents formally are told to do NOTHING: Just keep coming in to an orthopedic surgeon's office every few months for another x-ray, and wait to see if it gets worse."[104]

---

104 Hawes, M.C. (2010). *Scoliosis and the Human Spine.* Tucson, Arizona: West Press. Print.

Don't Try Anything Else

Not only are patients advised to do nothing, but they are discouraged from seeking alternative treatments or just informed that there is nothing they can do.

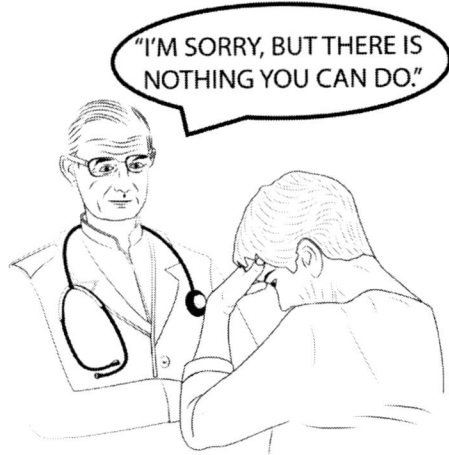

"I'M SORRY, BUT THERE IS NOTHING YOU CAN DO."

"If individuals insist on searching out help on their own they are treated to condescension and insinuations that they are being irresponsible by trying 'scientifically unproven' treatments and refusing to accept the advice of professionals who know best (e.g. Keim, 1987; Lonstein, 1995a)." (Hawes 2010)

Screening Leads to Surgery

Since screening has begun, there have been more scoliosis surgeries performed. Is there a correlation?

If the goal were to decrease the number of adolescents subjected to spinal fusion surgery, then why are so many patients being referred to orthopedic surgeons? Since screening has been mandated, the average curve for which surgery is carried out decreased from a Cobb angle of 60 degrees to a Cobb angle of 42 degrees (Lonstein et al., 1987). This was done as a means to operate sooner, rather than later, under the assumption that moderate curves will inevitably become severe curves. But, as Dr. Hawes points out in her book, "there are a lot more moderate (42° curves) than severe (60° curves) curvatures in the population." If one were to take a more cynical perspective, one could say that decreasing the average curve size indicated for surgery provides the surgeons with many more cases on which to operate.

Surgeons Would Be Put Out of Business

In the United States in 2009, spinal surgery to correct adolescent idiopathic scoliosis ranked second only to appendicitis among children 10 to 17 years of age.[105]

"...if proactive therapies were found to be effective, orthopedic surgeons would be put out of the business of spinal fusion surgery because there would be no progression to levels where such intervention might be warranted. (Hawes 2010)

According to Drs Martin, Pugely, Gao, and Clark of The Department of Orthopaedic Surgery and Rehabilitation at the University of Iowa Hospitals and Clinics, as cited online in a Health Advances article "Economic Impact of Novel Sublaminar Bands for AIS Fusion on Hospital Costs":

"U.S. hospital expenditures associated with AIS management surpassed $500 million in 2007 and have continued to increase dramatically in recent years. A recent analysis of adjusted U.S. hospital charges and costs associated with AIS spinal fusion surgery demonstrated that adjusted hospital charges and costs nearly doubled from 2001 to 2011, a significantly greater increase com-pared to other inpatient pediatric admissions, and likely indicative of a genu-ine change in hospital economics associated with AIS spinal fusions over that timeframe."[106]

Why isn't there more research on alternative treatments to scoliosis? Why don't insurance companies cover these treatments?

---

105 Weinstein, SL. "Effects of Bracing in Adolescents with Idiopathic ... – NCBI." 2013. 20 Apr. 2016. http://www.ncbi.nlm.nih.gov/pmc/articles/PMC3913566/

106 Cole, D., Ilharreborde, B., Woo, R. (2015) *Retrospective Cost Effectiveness Analysis of Implanet Jazz Sublaminar Bands for Surgical Treatment of Adolescent Idiopathic Scoliosis.* 23 Apr. 2016. http://www.implanet.com/wp-content/themes/theme-implanet/pdf/Health_Advances_Jazz_Cost-Effectiveness.pdf

Orthopedists Have to Do Surgery

There are many upsides to performing spinal fusion surgery as opposed to other forms of surgery, especially since scoliosis surgery is elective for most patients and arguably only done for "cosmetic" reasons.

"Orthopedists as a group relate the degree of satisfaction in their practice to the amount of surgery they get to do, and elective reconstructive surgery like spinal fusion is at the top of the list: High-skill, high-tech, very costly, covered by insurance, and no need to get up in the middle of the night to set messy fractures after car wrecks and suicide attempts." (Clawson 2001, Heckman 2001)

Some Orthopedists are Paid to Develop Techniques and Devices for Scoliosis Surgery

There is also the added bonus of money and grants received by surgeons from the companies that supply the instrumentation that they use during spinal surgery.

"Some scoliosis surgeons receive royalties and research grants from the biomedical companies who make the ever-evolving array of spinal implantation devices." (Shufflebarger, 2001)

What is even more alarming is the rate at which these surgeries fail and require further medical intervention in the form of secondary surgical procedures, known amongst orthopedists as "salvage surgeries." This surgery can hardly be called "elective," as patients experiencing extreme pain and impairment are often left with no alternative but to undergo further procedures.

"What is more, the worst that can happen is that the surgery will fail (as it does, often), and additional costly, elective reconstructive surgery covered by insurance (or the personal savings of desperate parents) will be required. Such 'salvage' surgeries cost $100,000 or more." [107] (Hawes 2010)

---

107 Hawes, M.C. (2002). *Scoliosis and the Human Spine.* Tucson, Arizona: West Press. Print.

Too Many Surgeons

Another major concern in the field of spinal fusion surgery is the large increase of orthopedic surgeons operating within the United States.

"The ratio of orthopedist to U.S. population has increased, predictably, from 1 surgeon per 110,000 people in 1941 to 1:25,000 in 1980, to 1:15,150 in 1999 (Clawson 2001). Surveys have shown that when the ratio increases to 1:15,000 or more, there is a significant increase in the number of operations being performed per 100,000 people, with concern that more elective surgery is being done than necessary." (Hawes 2010)

Remember, almost all scoliosis surgery is truly elective, this means the operations is not done out of medical necessity, it is done out of patient preference. Hearing of pressure to have surgery because there is "not enough elective surgery to go around" is very disturbing.

"An appearance of conflict of interest does not necessarily mean a conflict exists, and the vast majority of scoliosis surgeons undoubtedly are conscientious souls with a compassionate interest in their patients' welfare which overrides issues of personal gain. Indeed, leaders in the discipline have taken a strong stand in favor of the urgent need to establish and enforce clear ethical guidelines." (Shufflebarger 2001)

This is not to say that orthopedists or orthopedic surgeons are to be vilified for their practices, seeing as their advised treatment protocols are backed up by both peer-reviewed medical research and the insurance industry (that happen to fund said protocols). As Dr. Hawes also points out, one of the greatest contributors to scoliosis research, the Scoliosis Research Society (SRS), is comprised of several hundred orthopedic surgeons. Not only do they conduct research to better understand and treat scoliosis, but they also report issues within the field of surgical intervention for scoliosis and have more recently set up a council to look into non surgical treatments

Do Something!

So, if patients are instructed to "wait and see," what alternative is there?

Do research!

Research other treatment options, read the scientific articles, check the blogs and forums, read the testimonials, talk with the patients. Do the work that the medical community won't do for you. Become an "expert" on your own condition, so you are prepared to discuss the issues.

Take a proactive approach to your health care! Don't be intimidated by your orthopedist. There may be a conflict of interest motivating their disapproval of alternative, exercise-based scoliosis care programs.

Surgery is Rarely Needed. It Should Be a Choice!

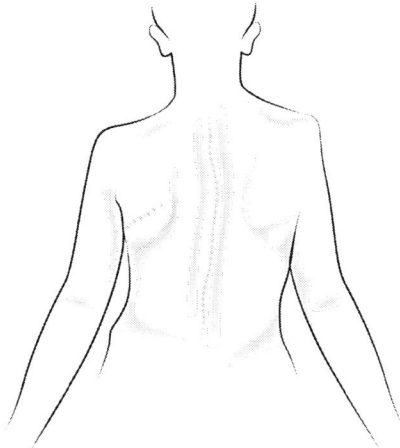

The prevalence of degenerative scoliosis has been reported as ranging from 2 – 60 percent of adults.

Rather than encouraging adults toward scoliosis surgery, perhaps the focus should be on establishing a better medical model. The better approach would be one that doesn't wait until surgery is the only option, but instead takes a proactive exercise-based approach.

Chapter 26. The Best Exercises for Scoliosis

A custom designed scoliosis exercise program can be a very effective part of a more comprehensive treatment plan for scoliosis. It's the type of exercise that is key! Exercise can be divided into two groups: isometric and isotonic.

Isometrics are a way to exercise the muscles while in a stationary position. **Isometric exercise** is experienced by pushing or pulling a fixed object like a bar anchored to the wall or floor or even another body part that is stationary.

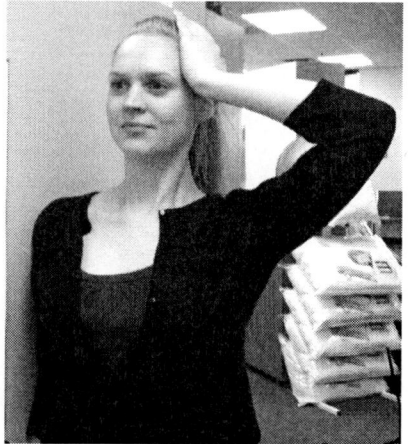

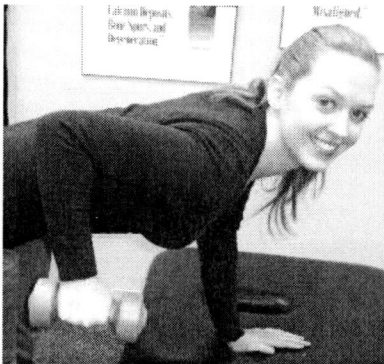

Research has shown that a muscle contraction during isometric exercise produces more force than a contraction generated by lifting weights. Isometric exercises can provide impressive results with minimal strain on the spine.

Isotonic exercise can be performed with free weights or with fixed equipment. Isotonic literally means equal tension. Isotonic contraction is when the tension remains constant as the muscle shortens or lengthens with body movement.

If you are unsure of the correct way to perform an exercise, please let your scoliosis specialist know immediately, as any exercise not done correctly will not have a positive impact on your spine. The type of exercise, body positioning, repetitions, and the order of the exercises must be individually designed for each patient. If you are going to put the time and effort into an exercise program to treat your scoliotic spine, be sure it is set up and followed correctly.

It is important to note that any complete scoliosis specific treatment program should include exercise as **part** of a comprehensive program of care. Exercise and stretches alone will not achieve effective results. This is because scoliosis is linked to a problem in the automatic postural control centers of the brain. Research has revealed that in scoliotic spines, the brain doesn't "recognize" the scoliosis spine as out of alignment. Therefore, it doesn't trigger the spinal auto-correction mechanisms that would fix the scoliosis. Exercises will increase flexibility and strength, this may minimize pain and discomfort and can even improve posture visibly, but the curve size will stubbornly remain the same.[108]

Exercise treatments and stretches for scoliosis need to be performed in conjunction with a specific focus on creating a stimulus that triggers the brain to recognize that there is an abnormality and to auto-correct the spinal posture. This stimulus must affect the body at a subconscious level to create any meaningful changes in posture. If posture changes are accomplished wilfully and consciously, as soon as patients take their attention off their posture, they will revert to the baseline posture which is supporting the scoliosis. In other words, any type of voluntary movement is overriding the subconscious automatic postural control centers in the brain and not allowing them to "learn" how to auto-correct the scoliosis spine.

---

108 Schimmel, JJP. "Adolescent Idiopathic Scoliosis and Spinal Fusion Do Not Substantially ..." 2015. 26 Apr. 2016. http://www.ncbi.nlm.nih.gov/pmc/articles/PMC4459442/

The most effective scoliosis stretches and exercises must be performed along with patient-specific, three-dimensional corrective exercises called "**neuromuscular re-education.**" This method uses the automatic postural control centers in the brain which are stimulated subconsciously. Patient-specific 3-D weighting (neuromuscular re-education) manipulates the spine and posture with necessary stimulus. Used in conjunction with customized scoliosis exercises, this routine can provide dramatic results by promoting a subconscious muscle response, both lengthening and strengthening muscles and retraining one's posture to assume a more balanced alignment to gravity. This results in stabilization, followed by a reduction of the magnitude of scoliotic curve.

All these exercises must be prescribed individually. based on size, location and rotational component of the scoliosis along with the age, flexibility, coordination, and stamina of the patient. Scoliosis is different in every patient and the best scoliosis exercises must be customized to promote the best outcome.

While the scoliosis patient is strongly encouraged to participate in other forms of exercise, such as swimming, team sports, Pilates, and yoga, they must not replace or inhibit scoliosis treatment or exacerbate the existing curvature. Be sure to discuss all forms of exercise and stretching with a scoliosis specialist.

Types of Muscle

For the person interested in a detailed understanding of muscles, physiology and why specific types of exercise therapy are so effective in treating scoliosis, read on!

Skeletal muscle is a form of striated muscle tissue (a form of muscle fiber clustered in parallel configurations) controlled by the somatic nervous system (associated with the voluntary control of body movements via skeletal muscles). It is one of three major muscle types; the others are cardiac (striated heart muscle) and smooth muscle (involuntary non-striated muscle). Most skeletal muscles are attached to bones by tendons. Skeletal muscle is made up of individual components known as myocytes, or "muscle cells," sometimes referred to as "muscle fibers."

Muscle fibers fall into two categories:

Type I fibers (slow to fatigue) appear red due to the presence of the oxygen-binding protein myoglobin. These fibers are suited for endurance.

Type II fibers (fast twitch) are white due to the absence of myoglobin and a reliance on glycolytic enzymes. These fibers are efficient for short bursts of speed and power. These fibers are quicker to fatigue.

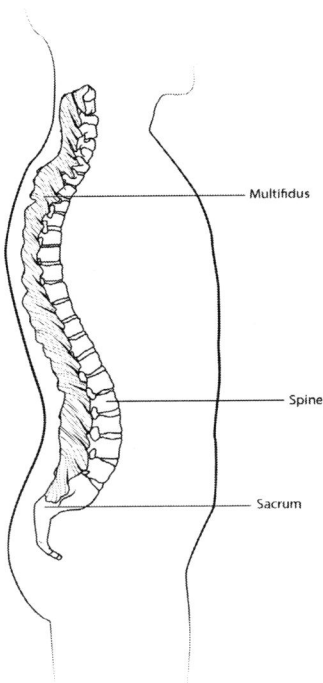

Multifidus

Spine

Sacrum

There are approximately five layers of muscle in the spine comprising superficial, intermediate, and deep groups. The deepest layers control the position of each spinal vertebra. These muscles are a significantly different fiber type than the more superficial muscles in the first three layers. The deeper muscle layers are smaller, only one to three inches in length and are mainly **Type I fibers** that are fatigue resistant. Studies have demonstrated asymmetry of these muscles (**multifidus muscles**) in people with scoliosis, and they are thought to contribute greatly to the twisting and tilted individual vertebral positions in scoliosis. [109]

Muscle fiber type dictates how a muscle responds to force/load principles. These deeper spinal muscles are not under voluntary control, and hence, NOT affected by standard isotonic exercise programs. This means that deep muscle groupings like the multifidi serve to support the body relative to gravity and also have the largest ability to alter the structural position of a single vertebrae.

109 Jiang J, Meng Y, Jin X, Zhang C, Zhao J, Wang C, Gao R, Zhou X. "Volumetric and fatty infiltration imbalance of deep paravertebral muscles in adolescent idiopathic scoliosis." *Med Sci Monit.* 2017;23:2089–2095.

Voluntary exercise programs for scoliosis like yoga and Pilates fail to stop progression, fail to reduce an existing spinal curvature, and fail to reduce the number of scoliosis curvatures progressing to surgical threshold because they do not engage this deeper muscle layer.

Spinal resistance training allows for subconscious involuntary muscle control to be affected, causing a change in the postural feedback mechanism that alters individual vertebral positions.

Spinal resistance training, using specialized scoliosis cantilevers, have demonstrated significant influence on multifidus muscles, causing less tilt and rotation of the vertebrae. The earlier a patient begins this spinal resistance training, the better the chances of permanently decreasing existing spinal curvature and halting progression.

So, if we look at the spine and how it functions, we can see that deeper muscles are shorter and more densely populated with automatic muscle fibers, ensuring upright postural stability is not lost. Superficial muscles are longer and cover greater distance, gaining mechanical advantage during movement. Therefore, posture, or "the spinal position" seen on x-ray studies, is mostly a result of intrinsic, deep automatic muscles which control the spine's position in gravity.

Automatic and not controlled by conscious signals, these muscles are not influenced by active conscious exercises, but react to specific stimulus (e.g. those that trigger a change in balance). Since the body has an existing "program" of how it aligns its center mass with gravity, and this program originates in the brain, then exercises which cause the brain to change patterns are very effective in influencing the deep automatic musculature that directly controls bone position. Neuromuscular re-education (by adding weight to alter body mass around the head, torso and pelvis) causes the body to reactively change its postural pattern and directs antigravity muscles to shorten and lengthen to establish a new postural balance.

By using specific x-ray and posture analysis, the doctor can measure the individual spinal units. This analysis can also demonstrate which portion of the body's alignment is furthest away from gravity, either the head, torso, or pelvis. A specific amount of weight is added to a portion of the body, causing the body's reflexes to reorganize the body mass versus gravity relationship. This reaction is subconscious. As the body reorients to gravity, it creates a subconscious new body image. If done correctly, this new body scheme will have less postural distortion, less spinal rotation... less scoliosis. After several weeks, the subconscious body scheme has been altered, and the patient will stand and move differently. Posture, x-rays and function will be measurably improved.[110]

110 Gaudreault, N. "Assessment of the Paraspinal Muscles of Subjects Presenting." 2005. 23 Apr. 2016. http://bmcmusculoskeletdisord.biomedcentral.com/articles/10.1186/1471-2474-6-14

Chapter 27. Non-Invasive Customized Exercise for Scoliosis

Some Popular Non-Invasive Methods to Treat Both ASA and De-Novo Scoliosis.

Scoliosis can be the result of both genetic predisposition and specific environmental triggers which are probably interconnected. There is no one approach, adjustment, or therapy which will work in every case.

Therefore, treatment must be customized to the particular, specific needs of each individual patient. However, there are key aspects of any protocols which are essential to achieve consistent, measurable progress. Find a practitioner who has made scoliosis their life's work – a scoliosis specialist. Start with a more conservative approach and then work up to more invasive protocols. In consultation with an expert, start with an exercise-based program, then advance to bracing if necessary. Only as a last resort accept surgery.

The first step in developing a customized program of care involves gathering information about the biomechanical function of the entire spine – not just the area(s) affected by scoliosis. It is an **axiom** that you can control the middle of a cord by moving the top and the bottom. By the same logic, it is important to understand what is occurring in the neck and hips – often the primary drivers of curve progression – in order to affect the middle of the spine.

It is vital to start with a complete history of the patient. Your doctor must have a complete understanding of the specific physical and environmental factors that may be aggravating your scoliosis.

- Leg length discrepancies

- Specific genetic variants in bone shape or development

- Areas of arthritis or spinal degeneration

- A review of all pertinent medical history including any trauma to the spine.

- Weakened muscles

- Poor balance

- Compromised lung function

- Location of your scoliosis and its severity

- Age of onset of your scoliosis

- Poor postural habits

- Activities that cause repeated compression on the spine

- A shortened spinal cord relative to spine length

- Postural instability or shift

- Hormonal imbalances

- Neurotransmitter imbalance from nutritional deficiencies or nutritional excesses (e.g. selenium)

And many, many more....

Standard Chiropractic Treatment (non-scoliosis specialist)

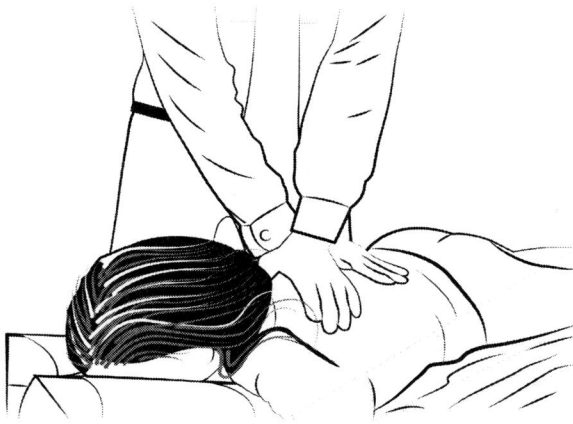

Chiropractic treatment for scoliosis typically consists of spinal manipulation, isotonic exercises and shoe lifts. However, research has shown that these procedures, when applied over a one-year duration, were not sufficient to significantly reduce the Cobb angle of a scoliotic curvature. Such treatments alone have been shown to be largely ineffective at significantly reducing scoliotic curvatures but can be effective in relieving pain.[111]

The CLEAR Scoliosis Institute

In the spirit of full disclosure, Dr Strauss is the vice president of the CLEAR Institute and a member of the technique advisory committee.

The acronym "CLEAR" in the CLEAR Institute name stands for Chiropractic, Leadership, Educational, Advancement, and Research. Established in 2000, the CLEAR Institute offers an alternative approach to the standard

---

111 Lantz, Charles A, and Jasper Chen. "Effect of Chiropractic Intervention on Small Scoliotic Curves in Younger subjects: a Time-Series Cohort Design." *Journal of Manipulative and Physiological Therapeutics* 24.6 (2001): 385-393. Print.

scoliosis treatment provided by the majority of orthopedic scoliosis specialists.[112]

Though malfunctioning brains and spinal cords are suspected as part of the root cause of idiopathic scoliosis, the medical community still focuses on the actual curve rather than on its root cause.

The researchers and clinicians at the CLEAR Institute noticed a crucial discrepancy between scoliosis theory and scoliosis treatment. They developed a treatment program that focused on "retraining" the brain to "learn" how to hold the spine straighter automatically, referred to as "three-dimensional auto-correction."

A 2004 study conducted by Dr. Mark W. Morningstar, a chiropractor and scolioisis clinician from Michigan, focused on the reduction of scoliosis by manipulative and rehabilitative methods. It involved stimulation of the involuntary postural reflexes utilized in a clinic setting and at home. The results showed reduced scoliotic curvatures in 19 subjects by an average of 17 degrees within a four- to six-week period with an average reduction in Cobb angle of 62 percent. None of the patients' Cobb angles increased.[113]

As reported in Dr. Morningstar's study, many of the proposed causes of idiopathic scoliosis are neurological. They include brain asymmetry, neural axis deformities, asynchronous neurological growth and central nervous system processing errors. Also, many coexistent neurological imbalances are present in scoliosis patients, such as visual deficiency and decreased postural stability (Feise, 2001) (Lantz, 2001). Therefore, the goals of treat-

---

112 "About CLEAR | CLEAR Scoliosis Institute." 2016. 23 Apr. 2016 https://www.clear-institute.org/about/

113 Morningstar, MW. "Scoliosis Treatment Using a Combination of Manipulative and ..." 2004. 26 Apr. 2016. http://bmcmusculoskeletdisord.biomedcentral.com/articles/10.1186/1471-2474-5-32

ment are not only to reduce the scoliotic curvatures, but to rehabilitate any underlying postural and neurological weaknesses or imbalance. [114][115][116]

The CLEAR Method of Scoliosis Treatment

The CLEAR Scoliosis Institute is an educational provider of certification and training for the **CLEAR Method** of scoliosis treatment. Doctors who provide this method must be certified by the organization. They evaluate a patient's scoliosis to determine what specific methods will successfully reduce and stabilize their unique spinal curvature.

To begin, they gauge how much resistance exists within the apical regions of the scoliosis. This rigidity of the spine is dependent on the length of time the curve has been present, the degree of rib deformation, and extent of vertebral rotation. The doctor using the CLEAR method customizes an isotonic and isometric exercise program combined with a neuromuscular re-education program that will challenge the intrinsic spinal muscles enough to effectively reduce and stabilize the spine curvature. Spinal resistance training equipment, utilizing innovative scoliosis cantilevers, are used to apply the different forces. These forces cause the spine to adapt in time and in need, with the result being a smaller and more stable curvature and, in cases of early intervention, the possibility of a complete elimination of diagnosable scoliosis (curves below 10 degrees).

The CLEAR approach uses spinal resistance training in conjunction with the principles of autonomic control of the spine's alignment. Some CLEAR doctors add a variety of other tools like bracing as an adjunct to their standard protocol.

---

114 Niesluchowski, W. "The Potential Role of Brain Asymmetry in the Development of ..." 1999. 25 Apr. 2016. http://www.ncbi.nlm.nih.gov/pubmed/10543585

115 Dobbs, MB. "Prevalence of Neural Axis Abnormalities in Patients with ..." 2002. 26 Apr. 2016. http://www.ncbi.nlm.nih.gov/pubmed/12473713

116 Catanzariti, JF. "Visual Deficiency and Scoliosis. – NCBI." 2001. 25 Apr. 2016. http://www.ncbi.nlm.nih.gov/pubmed/11148645

Principles that Should Guide Treatment Protocols for Scoliosis

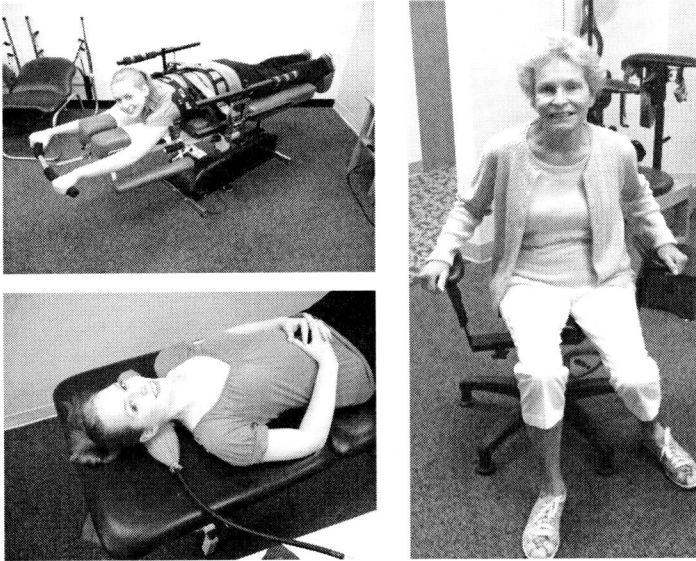

Figure 1. Eckard Table (top), figure 2. Cervical Traction (bottom left) and figure 3. Wobble Chair (right).

First of all, the best protocols operate under the premise that scoliosis is a complex condition. Secondly, all exercise-based programs need to have a warm-up component.

Patients need to warm up the soft tissues of the spine as a prelude to their exercises. What's the best way to warm up the spine? Move! Either use the mobilizing equipment or walk. Then stretch the spine. The **Wobble Chair** (Fig. 3) provides a good spine warm-up. It sits on a ball-and-socket joint, which allows the patient to flex her spine in every direction, promoting a full range of motion. **Cervical Traction** (Fig. 2) allows for active, gentle and, repetitive spinal traction), and **Vibrating Traction** uses a slow, relaxing vibration scientifically proven to relax the ligaments and soft tissues of the spine. Motorized therapy tables with belts that reduce the scoliosis during the therapy further improve the mobility of the most restricted areas of the spine (Figure 1). Warming up protocols encourage the intervertebral discs to rehydrate. This reduces rigidity. Now the treatment program can more easily affect structural changes to the spine.

The **Scoliosis Traction Chair (STC)** (Fig. 5) is a tool used to allow the spinal muscles to be exercised in a scoliosis-reduced position. The STC uses belting to pull the spine straight gently, traction to elongate the spine, and whole-body vibration to activate muscles.

The STC is a powerful form of scoliosis therapy, and the patient must be set up in the apparatus by a knowledgeable professional who ensures that the spine is properly de-rotated. Never use a tool like the STC without professional guidance!

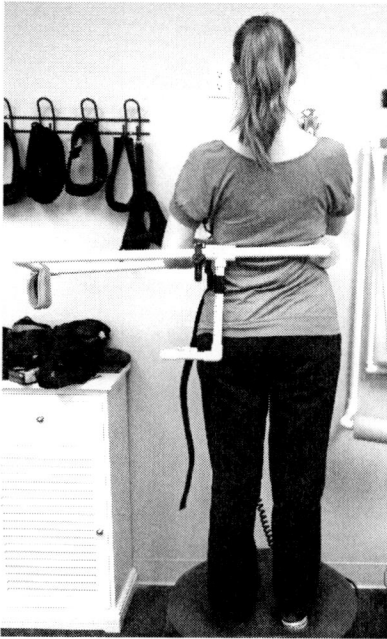

Figure 4. Neuromuscular Re-education (NMR)

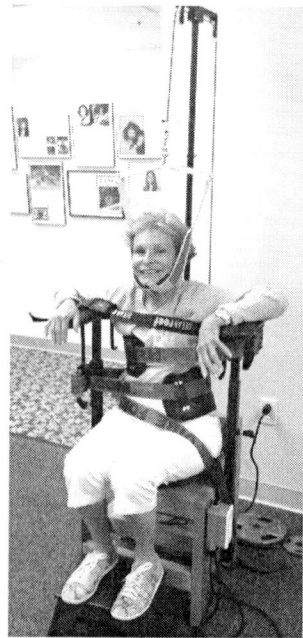

Figure 5. Scoliosis Traction Chair (STC)

Mechanical-adjusting instruments and a specialized therapy table enhance the precision and effectiveness of chiropractic care. These devices reduce the amount of force required to correct the spine.

In accordance with the most modern chiropractic protocols, almost all neck adjustments are performed with the use of such instruments, and the application of these adjustments are correlated with the information obtained from the patient's physical examination and x-rays. Treatments are painless, gentle, and applied with precision.

Locking in the Changes So They Last!

Immediately after the adjustment is completed, the spine is "set" in its corrected position to ensure the permanency of the changes, also known as **Neuromuscular Re-education (NMR)**. This involves spinal weighting protocols (typically on the head, torso and hips) and whole-body vibration therapy (Fig. 4).

If the NMR protocols are not followed, any corrections achieved in the spine will be temporary. The patient will simply walk themselves back into their original distortion.

The key procedures are assembled into a home-based program of care. Isometrics, isotonics, mobilizing maneuvers, along with body weighting, allow the entire program to be replicated at home with minimal equipment. The time for the home procedure varies from case to case, but typically will take one to two hours per day. It's a big commitment, but if it corrects the spine and helps a patient avoid surgery, then it's time well spent!

Follow-up Exams

Regular follow-up of the patient is critical for success. Once the custom-designed home program is either fully developed or well on its way, the scoliosis exercise specialist must again examine the patient and take a post x-ray to validate the effectiveness of the treatment protocols. This progress examination should evaluate all the findings evident on the patient's initial evaluation. Specific x-rays, which are necessary to assess correction, are limited as much as possible.

It's important to keep in mind that not all patients will show a reduction in the severity of the scoliotic curve, as measured by Cobb angle, within this time frame. This is because Cobb angle is a measurement of only two dimensions of the spine, and scoliosis is a three-dimensional condition. Before the sideways curve can be reduced or corrected, the spine must be de-rotated and decompressed in the other two dimensions. Treating a complex spinal disorder such as scoliosis is a little like reversing the path of a runaway train. It takes time to first slow down the momentum. Then more time is needed to change the course of the condition.

Home Spinal Rehab Program

The doctor and the patient need to have a frank discussion that emphasizes the importance of the patient's active participation in the treatment program. Results are not guaranteed – they are earned by patients who are willing to work alongside the doctor.

The traditional methods of scoliosis treatment, bracing and surgery, are considered "passive" therapies. The patient has the procedures done to them: the doctor designs the brace, and the doctor performs the surgery. Home exercise-based scoliosis specific programs of care, by comparison, should be considered an "active" process – the doctor teaches the patient how to do the procedures, and the patient does them. A small part of the protocols could be considered passive, but the effectiveness of these treatments on their own is limited without the involvement of the patient. Enthusiastic patient participation is the number one predictor of success.

There's a Role for Post-surgery Exercise Programs of Care

Patients who have undergone scoliosis surgery in the past may wish to pursue an exercise-based scoliosis treatment specifically directed at the areas of the spine that have not been fused. However, these patients should not expect any degree of correction, but rather purely symptomatic relief and functional improvement (e.g., treatment to relieve their pain, improve posture and improve their activities of daily living).

It is well established that muscular atrophy undoubtedly will occur in surgically treated patients. If the muscles responsible for moving the spine are inactive for long periods of time, they will atrophy (shrink), and because rehabilitation of the muscles is a vital part of any home exercise-based scoliosis program, the patient may be unable to maintain any corrections that are achieved.

All indications are that future scoliosis treatment will focus on the underlying neuro-muscular component of the scoliotic spine and not just the symptom as measured by Cobb angle. Proactive custom-designed scoliosis exercise programs in the earliest stages of idiopathic scoliosis will be proven to be essential.

Types of Scoliosis Exercise Programs

There are a variety of exercise programs in existence, each with a different philosophy and approach. However, all scoliosis exercise programs can be divided into two broad categories: those that are **stabilizing** and those that are **corrective**.

Stabilizing Exercise Programs

Stabilizing exercise programs aim to improve posture, reduce pain, and prevent the scoliosis from getting worse. These programs, however, do not reverse the scoliosis curve.

Examples of stabilizing exercise programs are (in alphabetical order)[117]:

CBP (Chiropractic Bio Physics): A system of exercise, traction, and spinal manipulation based on the principle of mirror imaging spinal distortions. This system was started in California by Dr Don Harrison in 1980.

---

117 Berdishevsky,H., et al. "Physiotherapy scoliosis-specific exercises – a comprehensive review of seven major schools." *Scoliosis Spinal Disorders*. 2016; 11: 20. https://www.ncbi.nlm.nih.gov/pmc/articles/PMC4973373/

Dobomed: This approach was developed in 1979 by physiotherapist and physician Professor Krystyna Dobosiewicz of the Medical University of Silesia in Katowice, Poland . main technique involves active three-dimensional self-correction of the spine and ribcage, with emphasis on the "kyphotization," or forward bending of the thoracic spine.

FITS (Functional Individual Therapy of Scoliosis): A system that includes postural awareness, myofascial release, gait training, muscle strengthening, side shift, and breathing exercises.

Methode Lyonaise: Originally used as part of a bracing protocol, the Lyon school of physiotherapy for scoliosis uses scoliosis-specific exercises, spinal mobilization, and training the patient how to sit in a corrected posture.

SEAS (Scientific Exercises Approach to Scoliosis): Also known as 'active self-correction', SEAS is a trained exercise approach to stabilize scoliosis. This method is frequently used in conjunction with the CLEAR Method to stabilize the correction achieved during the CLEAR treatment. The patient is individually trained in front of a mirror on how to unbend and de-rotate their scoliosis.

Side Shift: This system is built upon the theory that a flexible curve can be stabilized with lateral movements. Breathing exercises are included to expand the chest cavity.

Vojta: This method consists of stimulating specific points on the body to create "reflex-like" movements that lead to something like "freeing a switch" or "new networking" within functionally blocked networks of nerves between the patient's brain and spinal cord.

Yoga for Scoliosis: A scoliosis specific yoga based on the work of B. K. S. Iyengar (considered one of the foremost yoga teachers in the world). It has been developed by Elise Browning Miller from California and started in 1976. Sometimes called "Furniture Yoga," this approach uses aids like pillows, bolsters, chairs, and blankets to produce a customized yoga program to stabilize the spine.

Corrective Exercise Programs

Corrective scoliosis exercise programs aim to stabilize **and** modestly reduce the scoliosis curve. They not only improve posture, reduce pain, and prevent the curve from getting worse, but often can even modestly reduce the size of the curve.

Examples of corrective exercise programs are:

CLEAR method: One of the most prominent exercise-based methods, CLEAR is based on three steps:

1. **Mix** – "unlocking" the curvature from the original position.

2. **Fix** — encouraging the scoliotic spine back to a more normal position using corrective exercises and gentle painless specific spinal manipulations.

3. **Set** — locking in the modified, straighter spinal position by retraining the brain's postural control center to hold the new spinal position.

Schroth Method: Another well-known system, Schroth uses isometric and breathing exercises to reshape the rib cage and de-rotate the spine. Its goals are to halt progression of abnormal spinal curvature, and in the best cases, to reverse the curves.

BSPTS (The Barcelona Scoliosis Physical Therapy School): A well-known variation of Schroth, based on patient education and psychological support. It is often used with bracing and, sometimes, surgery.

Hudson Valley Scoliosis' Approach to Scoliosis Exercises

Scoliosis exercises REQUIRE a complete treatment program!

The best scoliosis exercise-programs take a combined approach, utilizing elements from multiple techniques. Hudson Valley Scoliosis uses elements from CLEAR, Schroth, CBP, SEAS, and Yoga for Scoliosis. Doing so provides us with more "tools in the toolbox," enabling us to customize each program to the patient's unique needs, and thereby deliver the best results.

The underlying principle behind our approach is that scoliosis exercises must target the muscles responsible for **posture**.

Scoliosis researchers believe that adolescent idiopathic scoliosis mainly occurs due to a malfunction in the area of the brain, called the cerebellum that controls posture. Studies have shown[118] that the brain doesn't realize that the spine is curving, and because of this, the body doesn't automatically correct the distorted posture.

The muscles responsible for posture are mainly controlled **subconsciously**. While you can purposefully stand straighter temporarily, you will revert to the original distorted position as soon as your attention shifts to something else. Since postural muscles are "automatic" and not normally controlled by voluntary movement, they are not affected by the traditional exercises one might perform while participating in sports, at the gym, or during an exercise class.

Our Scoliosis Specific Exercises programs are built from 5 components:

1. **Targeted stretching** reduces tension on the spinal cord and mobilizes the stiff areas of the scoliosis.

   During the examination process, areas of rigidity are identified. These areas are the focus of the targeted stretching. Shortened neural tissues can also be specifically targeted for stretching allowing the spine to lift and lengthen. Targeted stretching is used in combination with other therapies and is not a standalone methodology.

2. **Isometric and Isotonic (modified yoga) exercises.** These modified yoga exercises improve mobility, de-rotate the spine and strengthen the core.

   These exercises are designed to elongate the spine and strengthen supportive musculature. This acts to stabilize the scoliosis curve, improve

---

118 Herman R, Mixon J, Fisher A, Maulucci R, Stuyck J. "Idiopathic scoliosis and the central nervous system: a motor control problem. The Harrington lecture, 1983. Scoliosis Research Society." *Spine* (Phila Pa 1976). 1985 Jan-Feb; 10(1):1-14.

posture and reduce pain. These exercises are also used to de-rotate the spine to assist with corrective techniques. Isotonic and isometric exercises are effectively modified and targeted yoga exercises and draw heavily from yoga for scoliosis techniques.

3.   **Breathing exercises** for lung expansion.

Breathing techniques, aerobic training, and lung function improvement tools are used in conjunction with the other custom designed exercises. The breathing instructions help push the ribs outward to improve cosmetics and most importantly, improve whole body oxygenation.

4.   **Active Self-Correction** specifically targets the muscles around the scoliosis to stabilize the scoliosis and are performed as part of everyday activities like standing and sitting. Supports or devices are used only during the introductory training period with this method.

During active self-correction, a person holds themselves in a corrected posture during everyday activities. For example, a person who naturally tilts to the left due to their scoliosis would be taught to lift themselves up and to the right while sitting. Active self-correction strengthens the counter balanced muscles, which stabilizes the curve, improves posture and reduces pain.

The effects of active self-correction are very similar to that of isometric/isotonic exercises. The immediate effects of isometric/isotonic exercises are stronger, but they can only be done for short periods of time. Active-self correction, on the other hand, can be done for longer periods as part of everyday activities.

5.   **Neuromuscular re-education** trains the postural mechanisms to improve the scoliosis in a subconscious way.

As mentioned, our bodies are programmed to align their center of mass with gravity in a particular way. In cases of scoliosis, this programming is incorrect, which causes the body's posture to be held incorrectly.

At Hudson Valley Scoliosis, exercises are performed along with three-dimensional corrective exercises called "neuromuscular re-education exercises." Neuromuscular re-education uses three-dimensional weighting applied to the head, shoulder, torso and/or hips to cause the brain to adjust the spine and posture. For example, in a case of a lumbar scoliosis, a weight is applied to the lumbar spine in a way that causes the curve to reduce as a reaction to the weighting.

The weighting is done while the patient stands on a stability disc. The combination of correct weight, correct positioning, and correct balancing results in a rapid reduction of the curve size AND encourages the body to see the newly adapted posture as the new normal posture.

This stage is essential to the **corrective** nature of our scoliosis programs.

Chapter 28. Other Alternative Methods of Treatment

Is Acupuncture A Treatment for Scoliosis?

Traditional Chinese Medicine (TCM) therapies have been used for thousands of years to treat health problems. TCM is a system of healthcare that includes acupuncture, massage, and exercises, as well as herbal medicine and syndrome-specific diets. TCM teaches that health is dependent upon an internal balance of energy forces called "yin" and "yang." Yin represents slow passive energy in the body, and yang represents excited active energy. An imbalance of these energies promotes disease by blocking pathways, or "meridians," that allow the flow of vital energy, or "qi," throughout the body.

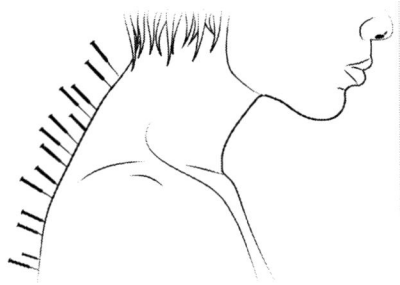

Acupuncture works to unblock this vital energy flow by stimulating these specific points in relation to the body's meridians. Acupuncture is used worldwide to treat pain and many other conditions. The most technologically advanced method uses a low-level laser (usually in the infrared spectrum) to stimulate the points, thereby unlocking the energy flow, relieving pain, and restoring function to that specific part of the body.[119]

---

119 "Acupuncture | NCCIH." 2015. 23 Apr. 2016 https://nccih.nih.gov/health/acupuncture

Cold Laser Acupuncture applied at traditional acupuncture points uses low-energy laser beams instead of traditional acupuncture needles to influence the flow of current at the treatment sites. It has been shown to cause an almost identical physiological response and brain stimulation pattern as needle acupuncture, except without any sensation. Laser acupuncture is used to treat painful conditions, headaches, arthritis, stenosis, muscle pain, as well as sinusitis and menstrual problems! Practitioners of laser acupuncture have studied traditional Chinese medicine and apply these principles to point selection. They aim a beam of light from a laser tube at an acupuncture point, stimulating the body the way an acupuncture needle would. The laser remains on the acupuncture point for 10 seconds to a maximum of two minutes.

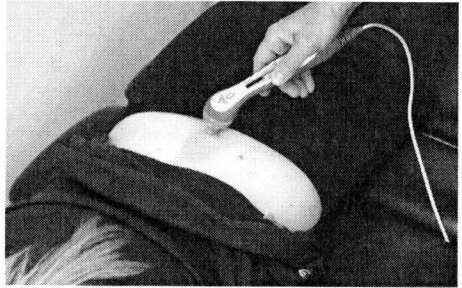

Since Cold Laser has gained FDA approval with an impressive 76 percent improvement rate, Cold Lasers are now being used widely in professional sports such as the USPS Tour de France and the National Football League.

Acupuncture and Idiopathic Scoliosis

Many studies have been conducted on the use of acupuncture; however, traditional Chinese medicine diagnosis involves syndromes defined by imbalances between the body's systems, such as yin/yang deficiencies, or qi stagnation, so results can be difficult to interpret in terms of western medicine. Because of these differences, very few studies exist on scoliosis and acupuncture.

One small 2008 study observed the effects of acupuncture on 24 girls between the ages of 14 and 16 with adolescent idiopathic scoliosis. Patients were divided into groups that received sessions of either "fake" acupuncture (needles placed at incorrect points) or real acupuncture treatment. Although no improvement was observed in patients with curves over 35 degrees, significant improvements were noted with the real acupuncture treatment in patients with curves that ranged from 16 to 35 degrees.[120] However, additional research is necessary to demonstrate the efficacy of acupuncture for scoliosis.

As part of my Master Degree requirements, I researched acupuncture as a treatment for chronic back pain, I was able to confirm that acupuncture is effective at relieving pain; it unfortunately did not improve the patient's range of movement or ability to perform their normal daily activities.[121]

At this time, insufficient evidence exists to conclusively prove the efficacy of acupuncture in the treatment of the pain associated with degenerative scoliosis, but it's likely it would be helpful. I think this is fair to say because research has shown acupuncture to be effective in areas related to pain management.[122]

Keep an open mind! No science can explain how acupuncture works, except for pain control. Many modern medical processes have not been subjected to scientific scrutiny. Surprising, but true.

Can Inversion Tables be Used for Scoliosis Treatment?

Inversion therapy has been marketed as an alternative treatment for scoliosis. Inversion therapy involves being upside down or at an inverted angle to take gravitational pressure off the nerve roots and disks of the spine and increase the space between vertebrae for therapeutic benefits. The process is

120 Weiss, HR. "Acupuncture in the Treatment of Scoliosis – a Single Blind ..." 2008. 26 Apr. 2016. http://scoliosisjournal.biomedcentral.com/articles/10.1186/1748-7161-3-4

121 Strauss, Andrew Jay, and Charlie Changli Xue. "Acupuncture for Chronic Non-Specific Low Back Pain: A Case Series Study." *Chinese Journal of Integrated Traditional and Western Medicine* 7.3 (2001): 190-194. Print.

122 Tan, Gabriel et al. "Efficacy of Selected Complementary and Alternative Medicine Interventions for Chronic Pain." *Journal of Rehabilitation Research and Development* 44.2 (2007): 195. Print.

called **"inverting."** This can be done by handstands or headstands, hanging from a bar with arms at one's sides, or with an inversion machine.

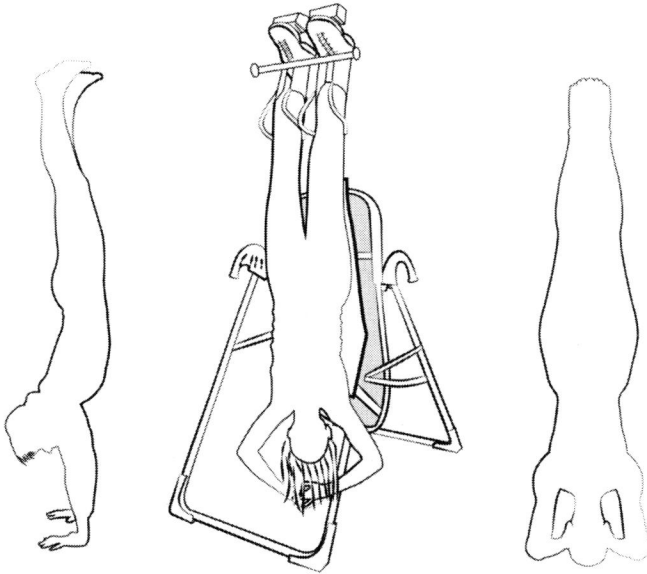

Claims

When the body's weight is suspended from the lower body the pull of gravity may decompress the joints of the body. Hanging by the feet, as with gravity boots or inversion tables, causes each joint in the body to be loaded in an equal and opposite manner to standing in an identical position of joint alignment. Inversion therapy is one example of the many ways in which spinal traction (spinal stretching) is implemented to relieve back pain.

Scoliosis Posture Correction from Inversion

Inversion therapy is promoted by some as a tool for posture correction. The increased blood flow to muscles may help to reduce back spasms. However, this will not reduce the degree of a scoliotic spine. Most current research suggests a neurological underdevelopment to be the cause of idiopathic scoliosis, that requires neuromuscular re-education treatment. In general adults must be very cautious with inversion as it can stress the body increasing blood pressure and intra-eye pressure of glaucoma as well as place significant strain on the ankles knees and hips.

Abdominal Strengthening

The *rectus abdominis*, or abdominal muscles, are partly responsible for the forward movement of the spine. Inversion tables can be used to perform sit-ups and crunches that strengthen these muscles. This will strengthen your core, but again it will not impact the size of your scoliosis. Scoliosis is not caused by (or as simple) as poor posture.

Research into inversion therapy and spinal traction to treat scoliosis is non-existent. Inversion therapy might bring temporary relief to scoliosis patients but should only be considered as part of a complete treatment plan designed by your scoliosis specialist.

Possible Dangers for Scoliosis Patients

While most cases of scoliosis are of unknown cause, scoliosis (particularly de novo scoliosis) also can result from infection, cancer, spinal degeneration, or other bony or neuromuscular diseases. Patients who suffer from scoliosis as a result of these other conditions should not be treated with inversion therapy unless specifically directed to do so by their scoliosis specialist.

Individuals with surgically implanted rods or supports could damage or loosen these implanted devices during inversion.

Remember, inversion therapy is not safe for everyone!

Khan Kinetic Treatment: A New Scoliosis Therapy?

The Khan Kinetic Treatment Device (KKT-M 1) is known as a "manipulator device." It's "equivalent to a similar pressure-applying device called **The Atlas Orthogonal Percussion Instrument.**"[123] According to the U.S.

---

123 "Khan Kinetic Treatment." 2015. 27 Apr. 2016 http://www.moh.gov.my/attachments/7489.pdf

Patent Office, the Atlas Orthogonal Percussion Instrument is
used to adjust a vertebral subluxation (dysfunctional spinal
segment) of the atlas vertebra,
the top vertebra in the upper
cervical spine).[124] This method
of chiropractic adjustment is
based on the 1960s teachings of
chiropractic developer Dr. B. J.
Palmer.[125]

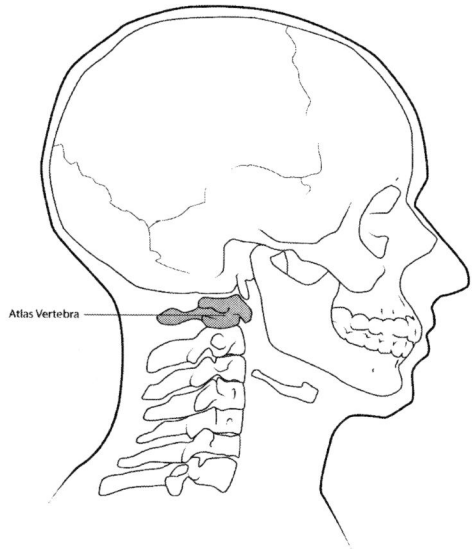

Atlas Vertebra

What It Is Used For

The device was invented by Dr.
A.H. Khan, who claims to treat
spinal cord injury, whiplash, herniated discs, back pain, neck pain, osteoarthritis, and headache. There is no independent research to back up
his claims.

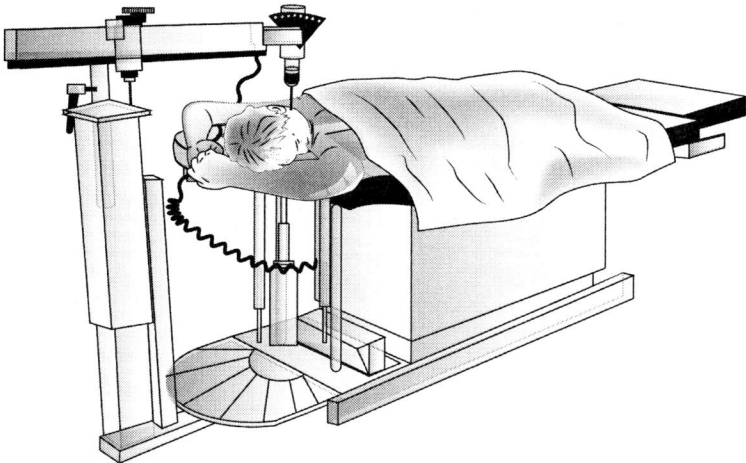

---

124 "510(k) Summary – U.S. Food and Drug Administration." 2016. 27 Apr. 2016
https://www.accessdata.fda.gov/cdrh_docs/pdf6/K060043.pdf

125 "Chiropractic: The Palmer Method (1963) – Chirobase." 27 Apr. 2016 http://
www.chirobase.org/05RB/BCC/11a.html

Editor's Note:

Dr. Strauss respects and uses upper cervical specific chiropractic as an integral component of a comprehensive scoliosis treatment program that centers around home-based exercise and neuromuscular re-education. While upper cervical chiropractic (as promoted by Dr. Khan) is a powerful tool to remove nerve pressure from the spine and spinal cord, it is NOT a complete scoliosis correction program.

Dr. Strauss is a past president of the Upper Cervical Society and has studied and researched this form of specific chiropractic in great detail over the past 38 years.

Pilates for Scoliosis

Pilates is a body-conditioning routine that helps build flexibility and long lean muscles and strength and endurance in the legs, abdominals, arms, hips and back. It puts emphasis on spinal and pelvic alignment, breathing to relieve stress and allow adequate oxygen flow to muscles, developing a strong core, and improving coordination and balance.

There are books and centers dedicated to "Pilates for Scoliosis" or "Scoliosis Pilates;" however, there is no research proving the effectiveness of these programs. Though Pilates can be added to a scoliosis treatment program, it is important to discuss it first with the specialist who is treating your scoliosis, as some moves may exacerbate your curve.

Because of the complexity of scoliosis, programs like Pilates – which generally target the body's core – are not designed to correct scoliosis but aim at stabilizing participants' back curves and reducing discomfort. It could be excellent when accompanying a custom-designed scoliosis corrective program, but inadequate if used in isolation.

Yoga for Scoliosis

Yoga's purpose is to create a balance in the body through the development of strength and flexibility. This is achieved with the ongoing practice of poses, or postures, each of which has specific physical benefits. The poses can be done quickly in succession, creating heat in the body through movement – as in vinyasa-style yoga – or more slowly to increase stamina and perfect the alignment of the pose.[126]

The poses are a constant, but the approach to them varies depending on the tradition in which the teacher was trained. Like Pilates, there are books and programs for "Yoga for Scoliosis" or "Scoliosis Yoga," but also like Pilates, the same precautions should be observed. There is no research to support its efficacy other than as a pain-management approach. Yoga will not correct scoliosis or alter its progressive nature. While there is a DVD called *"Yoga for Scoliosis," its design is not to correct the scoliosis, but rather to strengthen the supportive muscles, improve flexibility and to relieve any associated pain. You will notice when you watch the DVD that almost all of the students in the class are adults!*

Many people hope yoga will help treat or cure adult idiopathic or de novo scoliosis or even believe that they can treat their scoliosis themselves. The assumption here is that scoliosis is caused by weakness. This belief is based on a misunderstanding of scoliosis in general and why the spine is curving. The current scientific literature shows that electromyography (EMG) testing goes against the assumption that scoliosis is caused by weak muscles.[127]

The muscles in scoliosis patients aren't weak; they are misdirected and uncoordinated in terms of postural control. Postural control centers are located in the brain stem and are controlled subconsciously. What this means is that while one can stand up straighter through voluntary effort, an individual does NOT have direct control over how their spine orients to gravity.

---

126 "Introduction to Vinyasa Flow Yoga – Health." 2016. 27 Apr. 2016 https://www.verywell.com/introduction-to-vinyasa-flow-yoga-3566892

127 "EMG (Electromyogram) – KidsHealth." 2016. 23 Apr. 2016 http://kidshealth.org/parent/general/sick/emg.html

So, for example, when you consciously contort into a yoga pose, it does not influence the automatic posture centers of the brain. Therefore, these poses will have little to no effect on the automatic spinal muscles that pull the bones into a scoliotic curve.

These same EMG studies have shown that the very tight muscles on the outside of a scoliotic curve are actually attempting to pull the spine straighter. Therefore, there is every reason to encourage that type of muscle tightness. If you release it with yoga, you may actually increase the scoliosis.

Curve flexibility in scoliosis is primarily related to curve size and patient age. There are ways to biomechanically improve curve flexibility. By using passive stretching-mechanized therapies that primarily target the ligaments and discs on the inside part of the spinal curve, flexibility is enhanced in a targeted way. Stay away from releasing rigidity on the outside of the curve with general yoga.

That being said, yoga can be a useful component of a complete scoliosis treatment program. Yoga (as any other supplemental stretching or exercise regime) MUST be used in conjunction with a full scoliosis treatment program, and there are specific precautions to adhere to. **So, PLEASE READ the following precautions, risks and yoga moves to stay away from if you have scoliosis.**

With home exercises for any condition, it is always important to consult with your scoliosis specialist treating your condition before beginning any regimen.

There is much literature about scoliosis yoga and online resources with how-to guides, but this does not mean that scoliosis can be treated with yoga alone. It's important to discuss any supplementary exercise with your scoliosis doctor first to make sure it is suitable for you. Everyone's scoliosis is different; therefore, your yoga routine may need to be modified to fit your specific needs. It is never wise to attempt to treat your scoliosis on your own, even if it is a mild curve. Consult a scoliosis expert who shares your philosophy of conservative care.

Can Yoga Make Scoliosis Worse?

Many patients have inquired about the benefits and risks of adding yoga to a scoliosis treatment program. The short answer is that the benefits outweigh the risks... as long as caution is taken.

Here is an overview of yoga for scoliosis and how it fits into a scoliosis stabilization and correction strategy.

There have been studies conducted that suggest activities such as ballet, competitive swimming, and rhythmic gymnastics have significantly higher instances of severe scoliosis. Though it isn't clear what these activities have in common, it is believed that excessive and repeated hyperextension of the thoracic spine (mid back), or "backbending," may be the culprit. Backbends have a flattening effect on the thoracic spine, which leaves the mid back more vulnerable. An article about ballet performers shows an increased incidence of scoliosis in that group.[128]

Some yoga-for-scoliosis postures incorporate thoracic backbends and have the potential to aggravate a patient's thoracic spinal curvature. However, this doesn't mean scoliosis patients cannot practice *yoga*, nor does it suggest that they cannot benefit from this form of exercise. **You just need to proceed with caution!**

> *Read on for the specific poses that should not be*
> *a part of your scoliosis yoga program.*

A complete scoliosis stabilization and/or reduction treatment program will consist of the following:

---

128 Warren, Michelle P., Gunn, JB, Hamilton, LH, Warren LF, and Hamilton, WG. (May 1986). Scoliosis and Fractures in Young Ballet Dancers. *New England Journal of Medicine.* 314, 1348-1353. doi: 10.1056/NEJM 198605223142104. 1 May 2016 http://www.nejm.org/doi/pdf/10.1056/nejm198605223142104

1. An effective method of unlocking the apex of the curvature (yoga for scoliosis can fit in here nicely).

2. An effective method of reducing the size of the curve (that does not put any other area of the scoliotic spine in jeopardy).

3. A sophisticated analysis of the posture biomechanics and adaptive patterning that will yield a program of neuromuscular retraining that will lock the new reduced curve posture in place.

Proceed with Caution!

Let me begin by saying I have practiced yoga for more than 40 years and remain a daily practitioner. Having completed a yoga teacher training course in 1982, certified by Kripalu Yoga (SDF) of Napa Valley in California, I have personally practiced a wide variety of yoga techniques. So, I am by no means here to demonize or vilify yoga as an exercise regimen. However, I do think it is important for those with scoliosis to read this article before beginning any classes or doing yoga at home.

Though yoga is often recommended by well-intentioned fitness instructors and trainers, too often "scoliosis yoga" comes with counterproductive maneuvers that can make curves worse. While these moves are often very positive for normal bodies, some yoga exercises can be damaging to the scoliosis patient's progress.

Scoliosis is a peculiar condition. Each person will have a unique postural distortion.[129] Because of the complexity of curve type, size, modifiers, sagittal profiles and associated ligamentous instabilities or degenerative changes to the spine, it is not possible for a person simply to do "scoliosis yoga." For example, you may be improving one aspect of the curve at the expense of another area of the curve. A more realistic approach is to have a specialized

---

129 "Classification (King – Lenke) – Harms-spinesurgery.com." 2007. 27 Apr. 2016
http://harms-spinesurgery.com/src/plugin.php?m=harms.SKO03P

yoga for scoliosis program developed by a practitioner who is familiar with both yoga AND scoliosis.

When yoga is being done properly, no damage will take place, and the practitioner will be able to accomplish a specific rehabilitative goal with each posture. Yoga may have a positive effect on symptoms of scoliosis, but it will most likely not have any significant impact on halting curve progression or reducing the scoliosis spine curvature.

The type of scoliosis yoga poses that are best for you are determined by a complex equation reflecting the nature of your condition. Some movements may be contraindicated in your situation and be perfectly fine for someone else who also has scoliosis. No two scoliosis yoga patients are the same, and no one scoliosis yoga patient is ever the same twice. **YOU ARE CONSTANTLY CHANGING, AND YOUR SCOLIOSIS YOGA PROGRAM MUST CHANGE WITH YOU!**

It is also important to know that yoga for scoliosis alone cannot prevent scoliosis, nor can it stop its progress. You need to combine the scoliosis yoga program with professional specialized care to fully manage your condition and treatment options. A scoliosis specialist who understands yoga (or exercise therapies generally) can determine the classification, modifiers and level of curvature in your spine and then work with you to develop an appropriate pose selection.

BEFORE starting any exercise program – whether it is yoga, Pilates, isometric, or any other exercise format — check with the physician treating you, one who has a greater understanding of the principles stated above. If an unqualified doctor or yoga instructor suggests scoliosis yoga, please be cautious before proceeding.

Yoga Moves to Avoid If You Have Adult Scoliosis

After taking all the necessary precautions into consideration and getting approval and recommendations from the practitioner treating your scoliosis, you can establish a scoliosis yoga practice. But first, here are some poses to avoid or take greater care when performing.

MINIMIZE BENDING BACKWARD WITH THE UPPER TORSO

Bending a scoliotic spine backward is cautioned against because some research has postulated it may reduce the normal front-to-back thoracic shape (kyphosis). This "normal" part of the spinal shape works to limit scoliosis progression. You want to encourage this shape, NOT do anything to reduce it! By the way... backbend positions will not effectively lessen the rib arch. There really is nothing that can. Well, surgery (possibly with rib cutting and shortening) is the only way.

The concern that back-bending postures will flatten the thoracic spine and destabilize the area can be overstated. Take it easy and reduce the back-bends; in most cases you will be fine. If you notice any pain or aggravation of your scoliosis, talk it over with your scoliosis-trained yoga instructor.

Here is a list of the common back-bending poses that should be used only occasionally in a scoliosis yoga program:

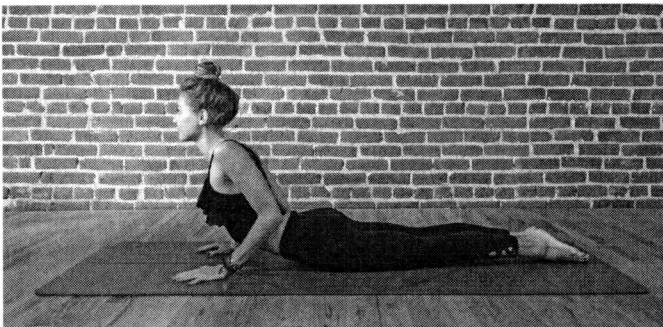

Cobra / Bhujangasana or Naga-asana

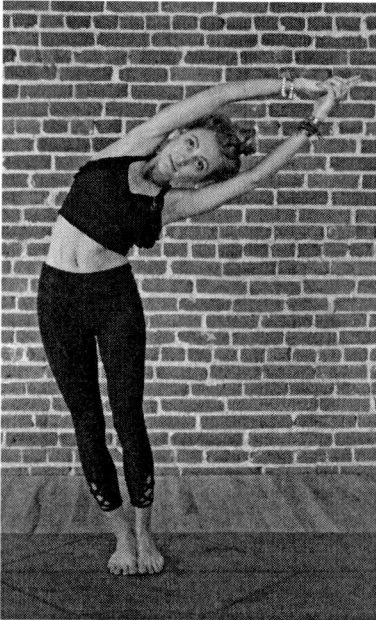

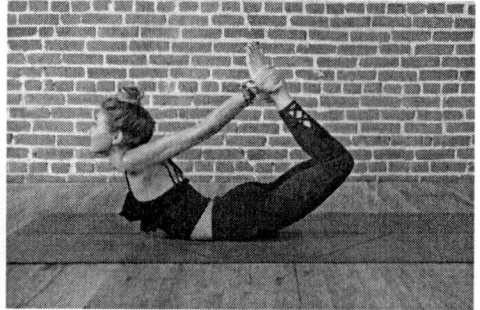

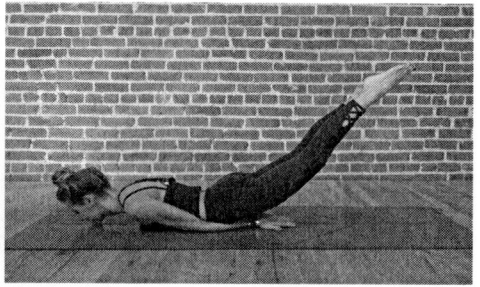

*Half Moon / Ardha Chandrasana (left), Bow pose / Dhanurasana top (right),
Locust / Salabhasana (bottom right)*

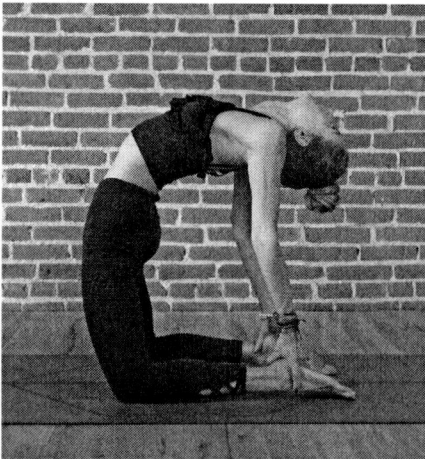

Camel / Ustrasana   *King of the Dance / Nataraja-asana*

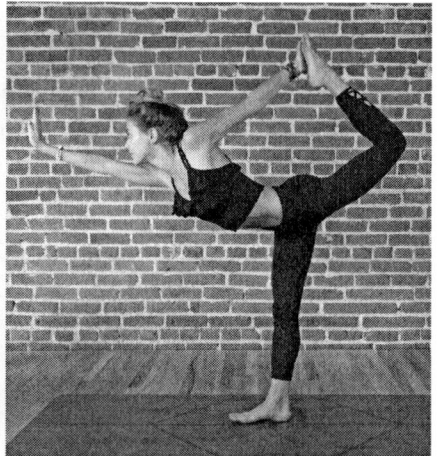

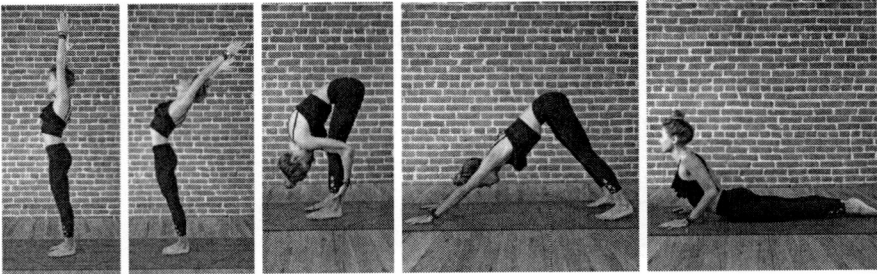

Sun Salutation

The back-bending in the Cobra or Upward Dog poses is a problem, so avoid these parts in your scoliosis yoga program. A Baby Cobra move would be a better option.

General Statement of Caution: AVOID POWER TWISTS OF THE TORSO AGAINST THE PELVIS UNLESS YOU KNOW IT WILL NOT AGGRAVATE THE RIB ARCHING.

The central segment, the rib arch, is enlarged as it rotates backward into existing curvature, regardless of whether rotation is to the left or right side. Patients with certain types of scoliosis can include these twists during their yoga for scoliosis program, BUT only to one side! Talk to your practitioner about these poses before including them in your practice. If you twist with great effort to the wrong side (or in the presence of a compensatory curve elsewhere in the spine), you are asking for trouble!

The Triangle should be avoided because the shoulder girdle is twisted against the pelvis, and the middle section must follow after the more comfortable side.

Other twisting exercises to use with caution include:

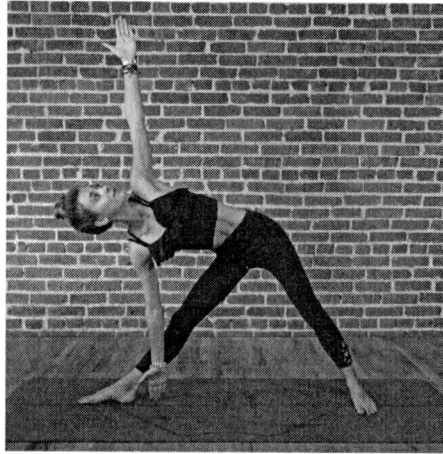

Triangle / Trikonasana

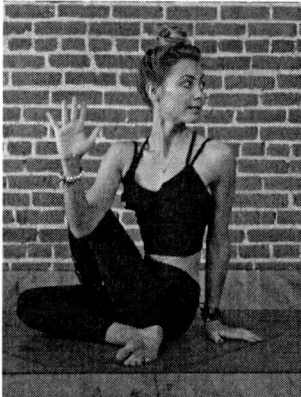

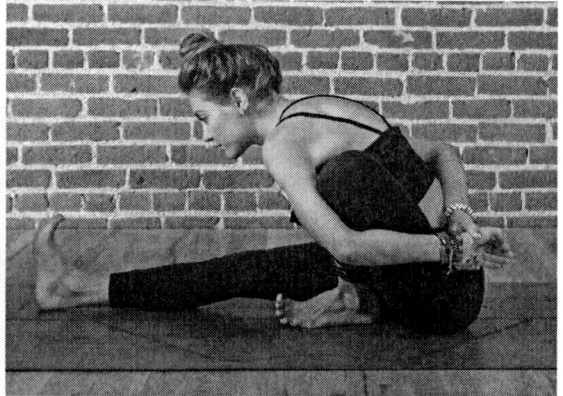

Spinal Twist / Marichyasana and the Seated Twist / Bharadvajasana

Trying to open up the main scoliotic curve between the thoracic and lumbar spine may improve the major thoracic curve, BUT at the expense of any other curvatures above or below it. How will you know that is happening? Would you be able to notice that the adjacent regions of your scoliosis were worsening?

Maybe... maybe not!

A scoliosis patient performing twisting poses to both sides would exercise into the existing curve and increase it. It is not recommended even if also performed in the opposite direction. This type of pose must be done only to one side, and if it is effective at unlocking the spine, it MUST be accompanied by neuromuscular retraining.

OTHER SCOLIOSIS YOGA EXERCISES TO AVOID:

Shoulder Stand / Sarvangasana

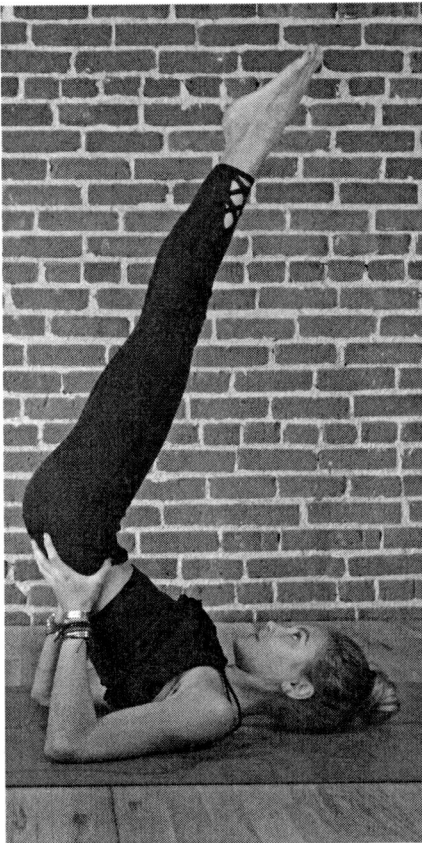

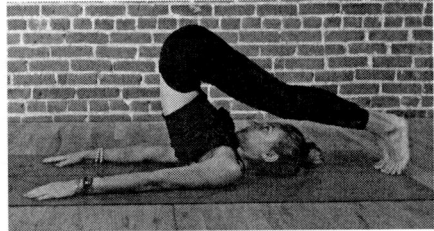

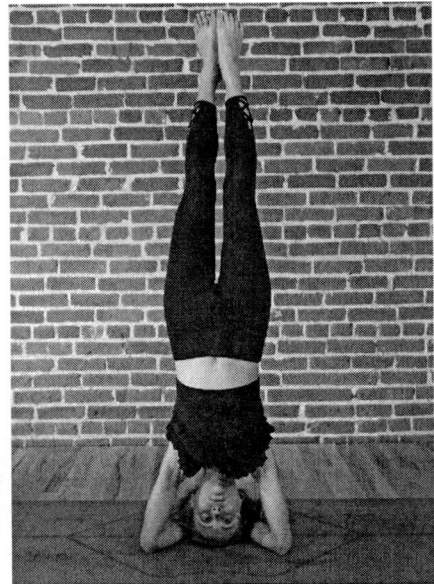

Shoulder Stand / Sarvangasana (left), The Plow / Halasana (top right), and the Headstand (bottom right)

In the supine Shoulder Stand pose, the head is bent sharply forward at the neck. This over stretches the neck muscles. It also will promote cervical kyphosis, a reversing of the normal shape of the neck. The whole-body weight is on the shoulders and may increase a rib arch formation.

An important part of any scoliosis yoga correction program is to work with improvement of the normal curvatures of the neck and low back.

Shoulder Stand will work AGAINST the establishment of normal spinal contours. Avoid it!

The Plow / Halasana

The Plow / Halasana pose affects the body negatively in the same way the Shoulder Stand does. By lifting the legs up and dropping them over the torso, extreme force is applied to the spine and upper back, working against the normal neck curve.

The Headstand

A scoliotic spine is inherently weak and unstable. Turn upside down and push your spine into the skull, and you risk destabilizing it further.

The upper cervical area of the spine, the part at the top of your neck, is often problematic due to ligament stress from scoliosis.

Doing the Headstand yoga pose will place undue pressure on these weakened ligaments. It would be better to perform isometric strengthening exercises to stabilize the weakened area.

Running

Short distance jogging and running are fine for most people with scoliosis.

Discussing fitness and exercise, the National Institute of Arthritis states:

"Although exercise programs have not been shown to affect the natural history of scoliosis, exercise is encouraged in patients with scoliosis to minimize any potential decrease in functional ability over time. It is very important for all

people, including those with scoliosis, to exercise and remain physically fit. The risk of osteoporosis is reduced in women who exercise regularly all their lives. Also, weight-bearing exercise, such as walking, running, soccer and gymnastics, increases bone density and helps prevent osteoporosis. Exercising and participating in sports also improve the general sense of well-being." [130]

Have a scoliosis specialist design or assess your running workouts. In addition to your running, a scoliosis exercise program will work to minimize any negative impact of running on your scoliosis and vice versa. It also can maximize flexibility, as well as strengthen your core and hip muscles.

It is beneficial to have your gait assessed for biomechanical issues that may need to be corrected. Orthotics may be prescribed or heel lifts if a leg length discrepancy is present. Use running shoes with good cushioning to lessen impact. You can have your shoes fitted at a running store to ensure the best support.

Run on grass whenever possible for less impact on your spine. Always warm up and stretch before your runs and cool down and stretch afterward. Stretching will help maintain spine flexibility and prevent joint stiffness. Pair your running with regular sessions with a chiropractor.

Can 'Scoliosis Shoes' Reverse Scoliosis?

Heel Lifts for Scoliosis

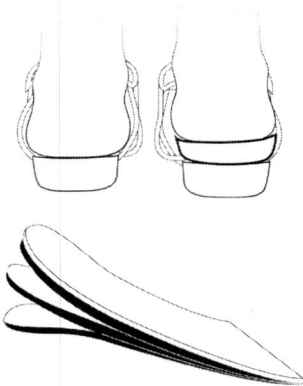

In the rare case that a difference in leg lengths causes or contributes significantly to a scoliosis, adding shoe wedges or lifts to the heels is indicated. A heel lift is a mechanical device which lengthens the shorter leg by a prescribed amount, thereby creating a more level platform or base for the spine. This method works in those rare cases where the short leg and only the short leg is causing the scoliosis.

130 "Questions and Answers about Scoliosis in Children and ..." 2008. 27 Apr. 2016 http://www.niams.nih.gov/Health_Info/Scoliosis/

While a short leg is quite common among patients with scoliosis, it is also common in the general population and a leg length difference should not be automatically blamed for scoliosis developing.

The whole picture of the scoliosis must be looked at before reaching for a heel lift as the primary treatment. Unfortunately, if the lift is wrongly applied, it can make the scoliosis worse. Other considerations are pelvic rotation, abnormal shape of the sacrum, the effect the lift will have on the posture globally, imbalance in the lower pelvis (the sit bones), and foot pronation. The calculation for prescribing a heel or sole lift can be complex!

Orthotics for Scoliosis

"Orthotics," "foot orthoses," "orthotic devices," or "biomechanical orthotic devices" are prescribed custom-made devices that alter the motion and change the pressure on your feet's weight-bearing surfaces. They allow for normal motion but limit abnormal motion. They can be prescribed to help correct problems such as excessive pronation, low arches, cavus, high arches and painful feet. They are also prescribed after some foot operations to help maintain surgical corrections.

By altering the heel height, custom orthoses also can be used like a heel lift to reduce the effect of a short leg, also referred to as a "leg length inequality." This can rarely be an underlying cause of acceleration of scoliosis

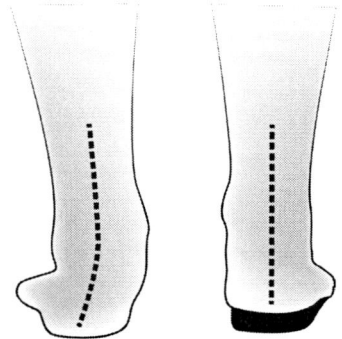

Orthopedic shoes, heel and ischial (sit bone) lifts and orthotic inserts can help correct posture in people who have skeletal abnormalities. Doctors sometimes prescribe specialized shoes and orthotic shoe inserts for people with scoliosis. These devices can help reduce associated pain and prevent further progression of the condition. Orthotics also can reduce scoliosis hip pain, scoliosis back pain, and other scoliosis back problems associated with adult scoliosis, if the pain can be attributed to a secondary orthopedic issue.

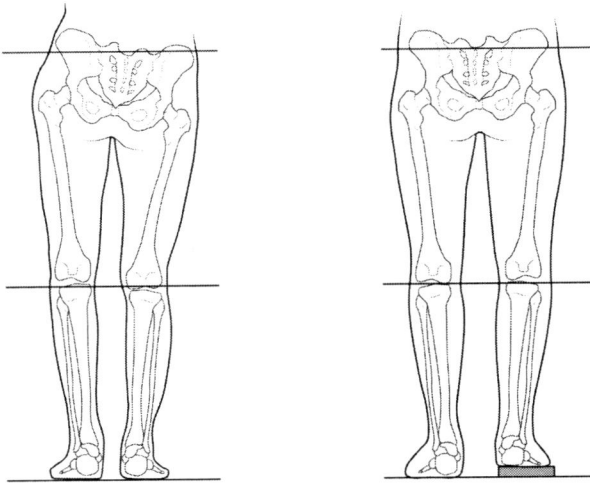

Research on Foot Orthotics

An article published in a 2001 issue of *European Spine Journal*, showed adolescent patients with scoliosis that had significantly reduced spinal curvature and improved postural adaptations (e.g. better pelvis alignment) after wearing shoe lifts.[131]

Orthopedic shoes and custom foot orthotics may prevent further progression of certain types of scoliosis and reduce back pain in adults with scoliosis. However, whether heel lifts can reduce existing spine curvature is still to be determined. More research remains to be done to clarify the use of orthotics in the treatment of scoliosis. By taking an x-ray with the orthotic in place, it can be determined how the orthotic is affecting the scoliotic spine.

---

131 Zabjek, KF. "Acute Postural Adaptations Induced by a Shoe Lift in ... – NCBI."
2001.19 April 2016 http://www.nejm.org/doi/pdf/10.1056/nejm198605223142104
http://www.ncbi.nlm.nih.gov/pubmed/11345630

> "*Whenever I write about mental health and integrative therapies, I am accused of being prejudiced against pharmaceuticals. So let me be clear – integrative medicine is the judicious application of both conventional and evidence-based natural therapies.*"
>
> **– Andrew Weil**

Chapter 29. Natural Cures and Scoliosis

Homeopathy and Holistic Practices and Their Purported Treatment of Scoliosis

Holistic medicine (from the Greek *holos,* meaning *all, whole, entire, total*) is a form of alternative medicine that considers the whole person (body, mind, spirit and emotions) in terms of health and wellness. Holistic medicine operates under the principle that optimal health is dependent upon proper balance in life.

Practitioners of holistic medicine believe that people are comprised of interdependent parts, and if one part is not working properly, all the other parts will be affected. This will create imbalances (physical, emotional, or spiritual) and thus negatively affect overall health.[132]

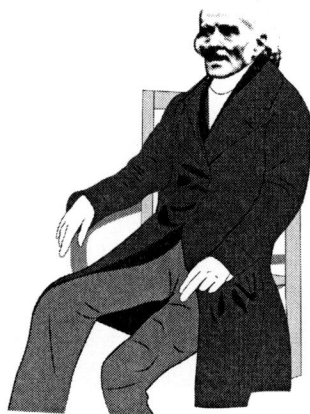

---

132 "Holistic Medicine: What It Is, Treatments ... – WebMD." 2012. 27 Apr. 2016
http://www.webmd.com/balance/guide/what-is-holistic-medicine

Homeopathy (from the Greek *hómoios* "like" + *páthos* "suffering"*)*, also known as homeopathic medicine, is one of the most popular holistic systems of medicine. It was developed more than 200 years ago by the German physician Samuel Hahnemann. According to his doctrine *similia similibus curentur* ("like cures like"), a substance that causes the symptoms of a disease in a healthy person will cure similar symptoms in sick people.[133]

Before we explore the use of homeopathy, let's set the record straight.... While many people swear by homeopathic remedies and use them regularly as their primary health care, the large majority of independent research has found most of them to be ineffective and their purported benefits implausible. So, in spite of the huge number of advocates in the general community, the large majority of the scientific community regards homeopathy as placebo care.

An Overview of Homeopathic Treatments and the Many Adherents Who Swear by These Unusual Remedies:

The National Center for Complementary and Alternative Medicine states:

"Supporters of homeopathy point to two unconventional theories: 'like cures like' – the notion that a disease can be cured by a substance that produces similar symptoms in healthy people; and 'law of minimum dose' – the notion that the lower the dose of the medication, the greater its effectiveness. Many homeopathic remedies are so diluted that no molecules of the original substance remain.

Homeopathic remedies are derived from substances that come from plants, minerals, or animals, such as red onion, arnica (mountain herb), crushed whole bees, white arsenic, lead, mercury, poison ivy, belladonna (deadly nightshade), and stinging nettle. Homeopathic remedies are often formulated as

133 "Homeopathy – Wikipedia, the Free Encyclopedia." 2011. 27 Apr. 2016 https://en.wikipedia.org/wiki/Homeopathy

sugar pellets to be placed under the tongue; they may also be in other forms, such as ointments, gels, drops, creams, and tablets. Treatments are 'individualized' or tailored to each person – it is not uncommon for different people with the same condition to receive different treatments."

The Status of Homeopathy Research

Independent research on homeopathy collectively has concluded that there is little evidence to support homeopathy as an effective treatment for any specific condition, including scoliosis.

It has been difficult to perform research on homeopathy because the key concepts of it are not consistent with fundamental principles of chemistry and physics. How would it be possible to explain in scientific terms how a remedy containing little or no active ingredient can have any effect. This has led to major challenges to rigorous clinical investigation of homeopathic remedies. For example, one cannot confirm that a remedy works when it has been diluted to the point that not even one molecule of the original active ingredient is in the bottle!

Another research challenge is that homeopathic treatments are highly individualized, and there is no uniform prescribing standard for homeopaths. There are hundreds of different homeopathic remedies, which can be prescribed in a variety of different dilutions to treat thousands of symptoms.

Homeopathic Treatment for Scoliosis

Here is a statement from a leading homeopathic organization on Scoliosis care.

"The selection of remedy is based upon the theory of individualization and symptoms similarity by using holistic approach. This is the only way through which a state of complete health can be regained by removing all the sign and symptoms from which the patient is suffering. The aim of homeopathy is not

only to treat scoliosis but to address its underlying cause and individual sus-ceptibility."[134]

In my opinion there is no scientific support for this statement.

Various Scoliosis Remedies from the World of Alternative or Holistic 'Medicine'

Editor's Note:

While Dr. Strauss believes herbal treatments may provide muscle relaxation, he does not think they correct scoliosis.

Herbal Oils

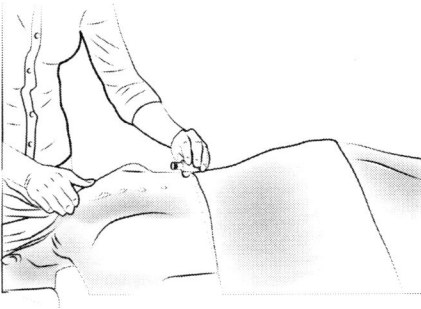

Individual oils of thyme, oregano, cypress, birch, basil, peppermint and marjoram are used in herbal oil treatments.

It is reputed that repeated application once a month will produce some realignment of the spine in cases of scoliosis.

Some believe aromatherapy combined with massage application will produce "a surge of energy" that is helpful. They believe oils deliver a frequency of energy, building on each other.[135]

134 "Scoliosis – Disease Index, Musculo-Skeletal – Hpathy.com." 2011. 27 Apr. 2016 http://hpathy.com/cause-symptoms-treatment/scoliosis/

135 "What Are the Treatments for Mild Scoliosis? | eHow." 2009. 27 Apr. 2016 http://www.ehow.com/facts_5006530_what-treatments-mild-scoliosis.html

Bach Flowers

Bach flowers are primarily used for emotional imbalances. There are 38 flower remedies that were
discovered in the 1930s by the late Dr. Edward
Bach.

Since then they have been used by many doctors,
homeopaths, and other healthcare professionals
around the world who have reported successful
treatments with babies, children, adults and animals.

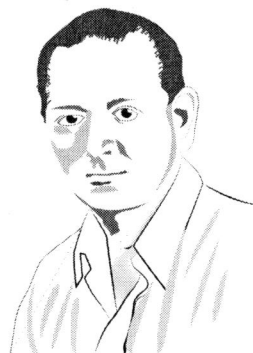

Rescue Remedy is the most well-known Bach flower. It is used to treat
shock. [136]

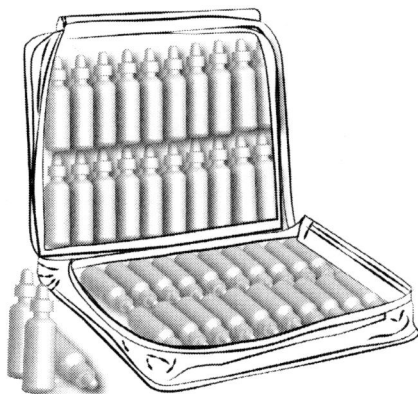

136 "Scoliosis and Bach Flowers – Alternative ..." 2007. 27 Apr. 2016 http://scolio-
sis.homestead.com/bachflowers.html

Chapter 30. Clothing Choices

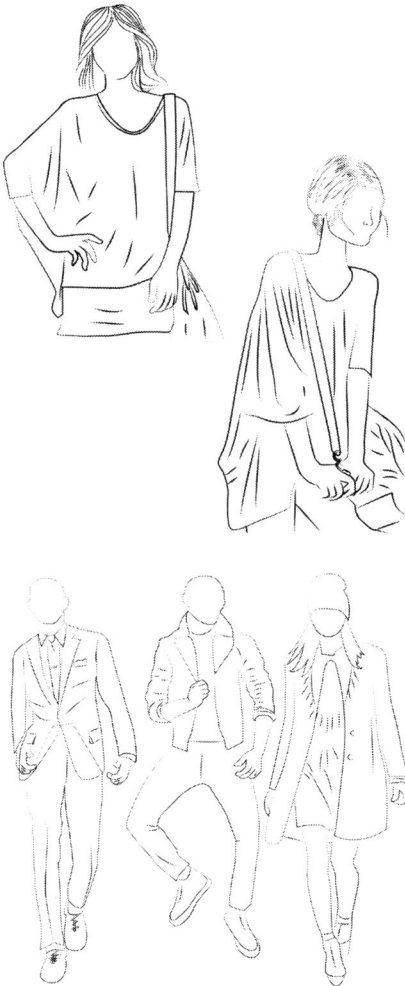

Scoliosis can cause visible symptoms: uneven shoulders, head held off-center, ribs at different heights, a shoulder blade that sticks out more than the other, uneven hips, one leg appearing shorter than the other, or the body leaning to one side. Severe cases will present with more visible symptoms.

Because scoliosis causes asymmetry in the body, ill-fitting clothing may be an everyday problem. The waist on pants or skirts may appear uneven, or shirts and dresses may not fit or hang on the body properly. Dressing in a way that makes the individual feel best and secure with their scoliosis can become a challenge.

One of the easiest ways to mask scoliosis is to avoid tight-fitting clothes. Tight shirts make asymmetry more obvious, and lopsided tightness is uncomfortable. This can even lead to aches by the end of the day.

So, if masking these asymmetries in the hips or shoulders is your goal, then looser clothing such as shawls, cardigans, hoodies, blazers, and jackets should be your go-to styles. Luckily, current fashion includes wearing oversized billowy T-shirts over tanks, and layering cardigans and sweaters.

If you feel too insecure to wear certain tops, a light jacket or sweater thrown over looks nice and can allow you the freedom to wear those items. There are many lightweight material options available. Even a Pashmina can be a quick and versatile option.

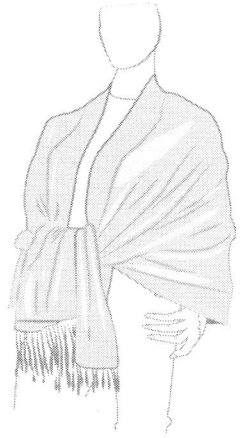

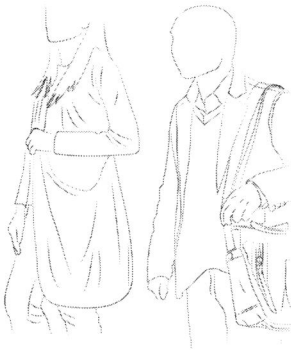

If it's a high hip that concerns you, then a nice wide bag can balance the difference. These do not have to be large or heavy, which will only cause pain over time. Many bags come in light-weight materials, so take the time to find the right one.

Smock, tunic and shift dresses are in fashion now, and compared with more-fitted styles, they offer coverage without being unflattering or boring.

For discrepancies in pant leg lengths, the best option is to buy pants that fit your longest leg the best and then hem the other side. This is an inexpensive alteration that a tailor can do. If you are frugal, doing the sewing yourself is a cost-effective option.

Dresses and skirts can look uneven at the hem for someone with scoliosis. A seamstress can pin up the hem to look straight while the skirt is on. Then later, she can stitch the new hem into place at a machine or by hand. It'll look uneven on a hanger, but that's OK.

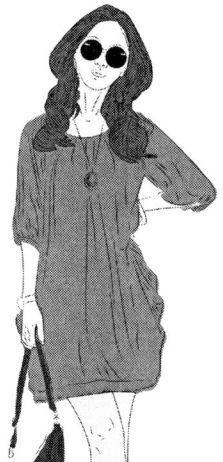

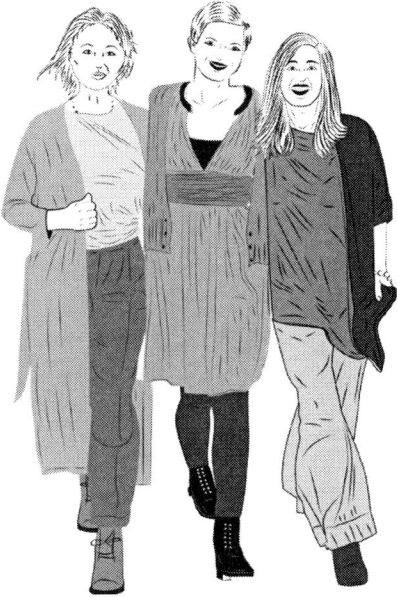

When worn the new hem will give the illusion that the clothes are straight.

The most important thing is to be confident in who you are and how you feel. Many people have scoliosis, including famous models, athletes and actresses (e.g., actress Shailene Woodley, actress and model Rebecca Romijn, Olympics track star Usain Bolt, cellist Yo-Yo Ma, and actress and singer Vanessa Williams).

You are probably more aware of your physical traits than others, so if you truly want others not to notice, then you must carry yourself as if there is no difference. People respond to confidence. If you carry yourself with self-confidence, that is what people will pay attention to – not your scoliosis!

Chapter 31. Can High Heels Make Adult Scoliosis Worse?

High heeled shoes have maintained their popularity for centuries, but are the visual benefits of wearing high heels worth the biomechanical detriment? What are the negative effects of wearing heels and can they make scoliosis worse?

As we discussed earlier, one of the many factors we take into consideration when assessing a scoliosis patient is Activities of Daily Living (ADLs), or the daily activities that patients perform at home, work, and school that may have an impact on their posture and indirectly… their scoliosis. There are various things that can impact one's ADLs and therefore affect posture. One such thing is the type of shoe you wear. But how could the type of shoe a patient wears affect their scoliosis?

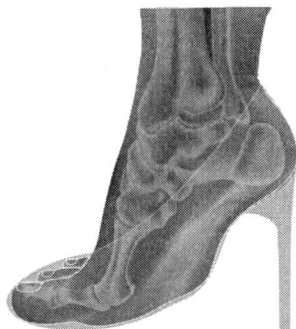

Bottom-up Effect of Shoes

The shoes we wear can have a bottom-up effect, meaning if they affect the feet or ankles, that can affect the knees, which can affect the hips, which can affect the back. High-heeled shoes, specifically, have a long history of es-

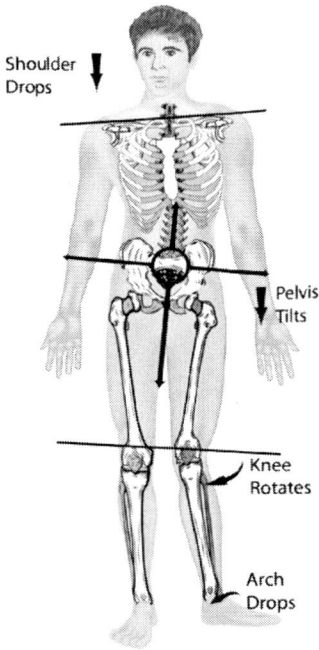

Shoulder Drops

Pelvis Tilts

Knee Rotates

Arch Drops

tablished harm. A study in Poland[137] wanted to test the harmful effects of wearing high-heeled shoes on the entire musculoskeletal system. The researchers evaluated the electromyographic (EMG) activity of the **erector spinae muscles** (muscles in the lower back) and pelvis kinematics of young and middle-aged women while they walked in low and high-heeled shoes.

Thirty-one young women (20-25 years) and 15 middle-aged women (45-55 years), with no prior back pain, were assessed while walking on a flat surface at natural speeds in three conditions: without shoes, in low heels (4 cm / 1.6 in) and in high heels (10 cm / 3.9 in).

In younger women, differences in the low back muscle EMG activity was observed at **initial contact** (when you step with your heel first) and **toe-off** (when you step with your toes first), with an increasing amount of EMG activity observed as the height of the heel increased. In middle-aged women, higher low back erector spinae EMG activity was seen during high-heeled shoe use. Interestingly, younger women had an increase in pelvic range of motion with high heels; however, this compensatory response was not seen in middle-aged women.

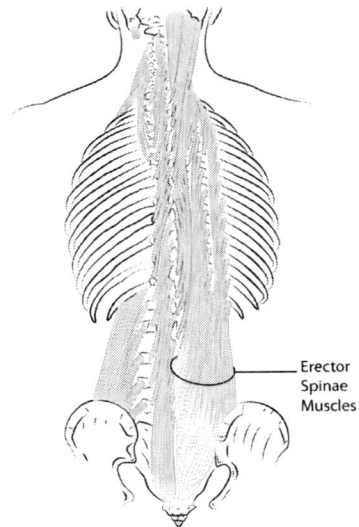

Erector Spinae Muscles

137 Mika A, Oleksy L, Mika P, Marchewka A, Clark BC. "The effect of walking in high- and low-heeled shoes on erector spinae activity and pelvis kinematics during gait." *American Journal of Physical and Medical Rehabilitation.* 2012 May;91(5):425-34. https://www.ncbi.nlm.nih.gov/pubmed/22311060

The authors suggest that increased lower back muscle activity from wearing high-heeled shoes could lead to muscle overuse and result in lower back problems. In addition, lower pelvic range of motion associated with wearing high heels in middle-aged women may indicate that tissues in the lumbopelvic region become more rigid with age and that the harmful effect of high-heeled shoes on posture and spinal tissues may be more pronounced with advancing age. Meaning, you may not feel the effects of high heels when you are young, but--as with most things--it will catch up with you as you get older.

Forward Head Posture

One reason so many people continue to wear high heels, despite the obvious pain and other adverse effects, is the belief that they make one's appearance more attractive. Many people claim that high heels improve their posture — that they stand straighter or taller as they are forced to balance in heels. If we take a look at the images below, the body does adjust to keep balanced, but not necessarily in the way most people would think.

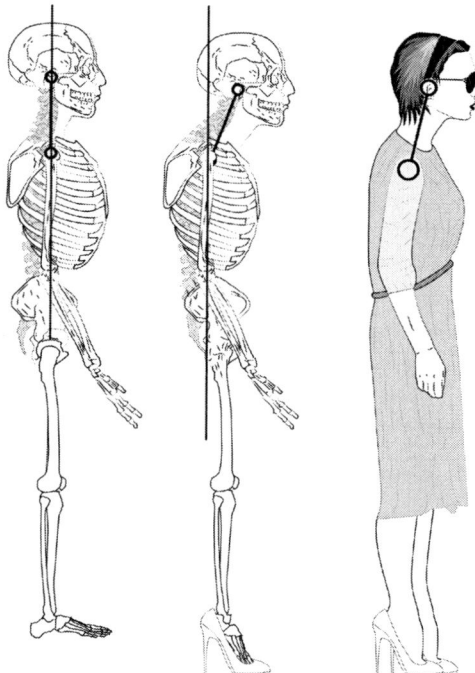

The effects of this altered posture over time can lead to forward head posture (pictured above), a Dowager's hump, kyphosis, and a flattening of the
lower back. Many of these conditions already accompany scoliosis.

Arthritis and High Heel Shoes

Osteoarthritis is a type of arthritis caused by wear and tear on joints. It is
the most common form of arthritis and is not associated with any underlying disease like orther forms of arthritis. Knee osteoarthritis is more common in women than men and is also a leading cause of disability. To identify the cause of this discrepancy, researchers observed 14 healthy females
while they walked in 3.8 cm (1.5 in) flat athletic shoes, and 8.3 cm (3.3 in)
heeled shoes with and without a 20 percent body weight vest. They found
that at a typical walking speeds:

- Knee flexion angle at heel-strike & **midstance** increased with increasing heel height
  & weight.

- Maximum knee extension moment during
  loading response_decreased with added
  weight.

- Maximum knee extension moment during
  terminal stance_decreased with heel height.

Knee Adduction
Moment

- Maximum **knee adduction** moments increased with heel height.

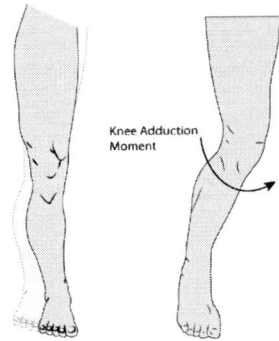

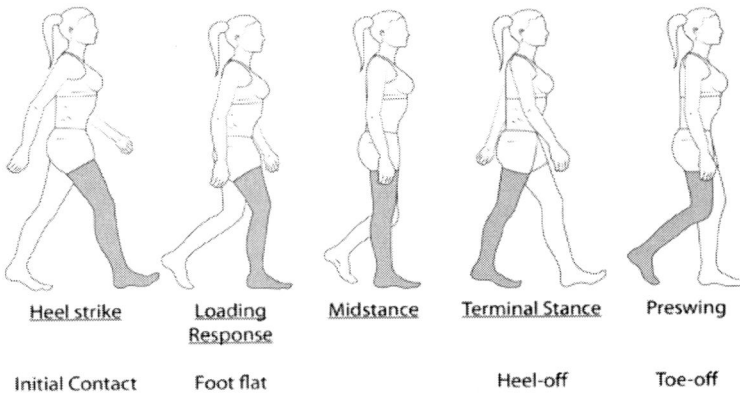

Heel strike	Loading Response	Midstance	Terminal Stance	Preswing
Initial Contact	Foot flat		Heel-off	Toe-off

Many of the changes observed with increasing heel height and weight were similar to those seen with aging and osteoarthritis progression. The researchers suggest that high-heel use, especially when combined with increased weight, may contribute to increased risk of osteoarthritis in women.

A similar study[138] from 2014 collected data about participant's self-reported footwear to assess specific shoe use per decade of life. With this they identified persistent users of certain footwear (i.e. heel height, sole thickness or hardness) from early adulthood.

They found that those who frequently wore women's high-heeled and narrow heeled shoes during early adulthood displayed negative associations with both knee and hip osteoarthritis. Those who persistently wore narrow heeled shoes were associated with less risk of osteoarthritis. Further analysis suggested that women with hip osteoarthritis may have stopped wearing high- and narrow-heeled footwear to reduce hip pain in early adulthood.

Another study from 2013 simulated **Heel strike, Midstance** and **Toe-off** to assess the biomechanical response of high-heeled shoe walking.[139]

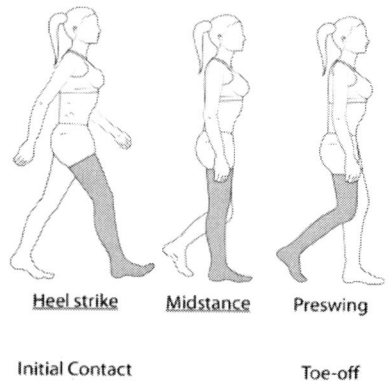

Heel strike   Midstance   Preswing

Initial Contact   Toe-off

They found that:

- Contact pressure at all the metatarsophalangeal (MTP) joints (joints between the metatarsal bones of the foot and the proximal bones of the toes) intensified and reached their maximum during **Toe-off.**

---

138 McWilliams DF, Muthuri S, Muir KR, Maciewicz RA, Zhang W, Doherty M. "Self-reported adult footwear and the risks of lower limb osteoarthritis: the GOAL case control study." *BMC Musculoskeletal Disorders.* 2014 Sep 20;15:308. http://www.ncbi.nlm.nih.gov/pubmed/25240981

139 Titchenal MR, Asay JL, Favre J, Andriacchi TP, Chu CR." Effects of high heel wear and increased weight on the knee during walking." *Journal of Orthopedic Research.* 2015 Mar;33(3):405-11. https://www.ncbi.nlm.nih.gov/pubmed/25532875

- The first MTP joint bent the most.

- The first and fifth MTP joints had larger movements of all the joints, indicating that these joints bend more significantly from the toe box restraint during movement.

- The top of foot's contact pressure at the first toe increased by four times from **Heel strike** to **Toe-off.**

This study demonstrates the intense amount of pressure and strain that walking in high-heels puts on the joints of the feet that leads to many different bone and joint ailments over time.

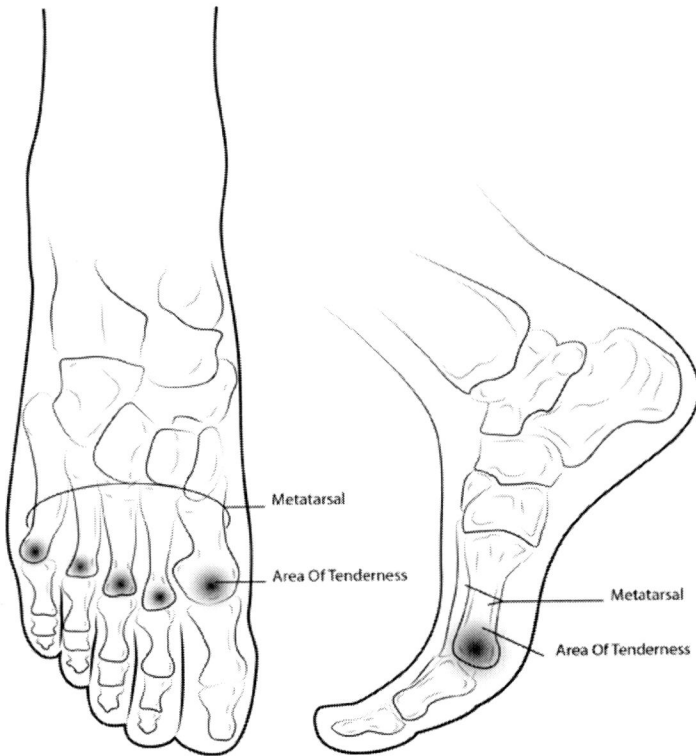

Metatarsal

Area Of Tenderness

Metatarsal

Area Of Tenderness

So, Which Is Best? High, Medium or Flat?

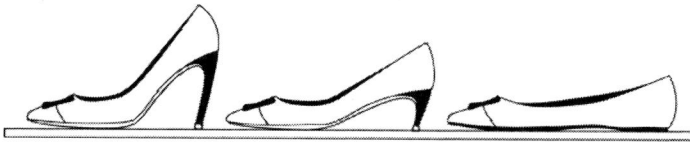

As it turns out, high heels aren't the only problem. A study from South Korea[140] aimed to determine the most appropriate heel height for shoes by measuring the displacement of the center of pressure and changes in the distribution of foot pressure after walking in flat (0.5 cm / 0.2 in), middle-heeled (4 cm / 1.6 in), and high-heeled (9 cm / 3.5 in) shoes for 1 hour. Fifteen healthy women wore shoes with heels of each height in a random order. The foot pressure and displacement of the center of pressure before and after walking in a typical setting for 1 hour were assessed. They found:

Both flat and high-heeled shoes had adverse effects on the body. **Middle-heeled shoes (less than 2 in) are preferable** to both flat shoes (less than 1 in) and high-heeled (3.5 in or larger) shoes for the health and comfort of the feet.

So, Will Wearing High Heels Make Scoliosis Worse?

Though research consistently displays the negative effects of high-heel use on posture and joint health, there has yet to be a study on how they affect scoliosis. There has been research[141] indicating that spine alignment might affect the control of heel, ankle and toe rockers in the ankle-foot complex. When patients ask what they can personally do differently to help their sco-

---

140 Ko DY, Lee HS. "The Changes of COP and Foot Pressure after One Hour's Walking Wearing High-heeled and Flat Shoes." *Journal of Physical Therapy Science.* 2013 Oct;25(10):1309-12. https://www.ncbi.nlm.nih.gov/pubmed/24259782

141 Chern JS, Kao CC, Lai PL, Lung CW, Chen WJ. "Severity of spine malalignment on center of pressure progression during level walking in subjects with adolescent idiopathic scoliosis." —NCBI. 2014. https://www.ncbi.nlm.nih.gov/pubmed/25571336

liosis, based on these findings, it's safe to suggest that to decrease or eliminate high-heel use certainly can't hurt.

However, one can understand that to ask a patient to completely do away with high heels might be asking too much. I certainly would discourage ANYONE from wearing high heels for 8 or more hours per day.

But is there any amount of research or data that can convince people to not wear high heels ?

NOW IT'S TIME TO TAKE ACTION!

Now that you have read to the end of this book, let me return to the basic issue we discussed at the beginning: do you want to eliminate pain, stabilize – and possibly even reduce – your adult scoliosis without pain pills, or even worse, painful, potentially disabling surgery?

Of course you do!

And I want you to act on your newly-gained knowledge to improve your life. Countless adult scoliosis sufferers have experienced relief from the pain, disability, fear, and poor self-image that often accompany scoliosis. You can be one of them.

Let me recap what you face — and the path ahead for you.

The 4 biggest concerns for adult scoliosis sufferers

- **Pain**: Though it is rare for scoliosis to cause pain in adolescence, pain is a common symptom of adult scoliosis.

  One of our patients recalls the sudden and unexpected onset of pain she experienced as an adult after having no pain when she was younger:

  Wendy cried herself to sleep at night because she was in so much pain. For 30 years, Wendy was told that all she could do was manage pain and remained dependent on pain medicine. After treatment with us, her outlook changed radically.

  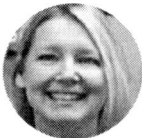
  "I experienced more pain relief in one week than I had experienced in 30 years from other treatments. It gave me power to take care of myself."

  Can you identify with her situation? If not, could this be you in 10 years if your curves progress? How about in 20 years or 30 years?

- **Disability**: As scoliosis patients become older, the likelihood of disability increases.

One Hudson Valley Scoliosis patient had such severe scoliosis that she could not walk and was confined to her bed. She was without any freedom and independence. But after just 6 weeks, she was able to walk and move again without any pain or discomfort:

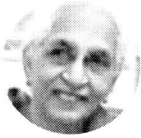

"After Dr. Strauss started my therapy, my back pain was gone within 6 weeks. I can walk well now."

- **Progression**: When you do not receive treatment for scoliosis and simply "watch and wait," you are vulnerable to the likely outcome that your curve will get much worse over time.

- **Aesthetics**: While pain, disability, and the progression of your curves are the most serious and urgent results of adult scoliosis, the way that you look when you go about your daily live is a very real and important consideration for scoliosis sufferers.

Research shows that even if the curve can only be reduced 15-20%, significant postural improvement is still very possible

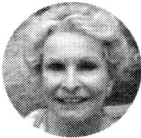

"I hated the way I was different. My friends were always asking me if I was in pain because my hip was sticking out to the side when I walked. Yes, I was in some pain, but I didn't want anyone to notice, but they all did."

Let me say this again: There is something you can do about the progression of your adult scoliosis.

You no longer have to live with the hopelessness, fear, uncertainty, pain, or disability that accompanies your scoliosis prognosis. And you don't have to live with the poor options with which you've been presented to either "watch and wait," have a major spine surgery, or wear an uncomfortable, ineffective, and conspicuous "old technology" back brace.

There is something you can do about the progression of your adult scoliosis. There is a solution besides waiting and watching your curves get worse or undergoing risky and spine surgery.

Why would an adult seek out care for scoliosis? Let me restate the Top 5 benefits of scoliosis specific custom designed exercise-based programs for adult scoliosis:

1. **Reduction or elimination of curve progression AND significant postural change with improved cosmetic appearance.** Yes! It is often possible to have curve reduction, even in adult scoliosis, and you are very likely to see substantial postural improvement!

2. **Gives patients control over their condition.** Scoliosis sufferers can finally be done with that feeling of hopelessness and helplessness for good, because with this type of care plan they know that they hold the power for real and lasting change.

3. **More lung capacity and more room for organs.** Many scoliosis sufferers do not realize the effect their condition has on their lung capacity and organ position. Once they begin to see improvement from their treatment, they can't believe the improvement in comfort and health that they feel.

4. **More energy.** Many of our patients have reported more energy to do the things they love to do such as spend time with their family and friends, be independent, and have enjoyable and productive work lives.

5. **Relief or reduced chance of future pain, disability, or deteriorated aesthetics.** This is the primary concern for scoliosis sufferers, especially for adult patients.

What should you look for in an Adult's Exercise based Program

1. **Effective.** Custom-designed home-based exercise programs have been effective for thousands of scoliosis patients worldwide.

2. **Treats the cause, not the symptom.** The reason custom-designed home-based exercise programs work is because they address the root of the problem by retraining muscle memory and strengthening the muscles of the body that work to support and correct posture.

3. **An alternative to medicine.** Over the course of many years on pain medicine, the cost is exorbitant and the toll on your health even greater. Most importantly, in the end, what do you have to show for it? No change or improvement of your condition — just a mask over the pain and curve that still exists under the surface and is continuing to progress over time.

4. **Custom treatment plan.** There are many variables to consider, including the shape and location of the scoliosis, curve size, postural changes, flexibility, presence of osteoporosis, balance, level of pain experienced, age of the patient, and plenty of other factors. That's why the custom-designed home-based exercise program protocols are different for each patient.

5. **No risk.** Unlike risky and dangerous surgery, you have nothing to lose by trying a custom designed home-based exercise programs. We have seen case after case of the treatment improving the condition and quality of life for patients of all ages. But if it does not work for you, you are not left with a lifelong handicap or chronic pain that can be the result of surgery.

Now It's Your Turn!

At the end of this chapter you will see the testimonials of many scoliosis sufferers who have had significant improvements in their conditions after exercise-based scoliosis treatment.

Why not let that be your story?

You're Standing at a Crossroads... Which Way Will You Choose?

You have three options.

1. Your first option is to do nothing. This takes you down a tortuous road of pain, frustration and embarrassment as you try to deal with your scoliosis instead of fighting it and getting your life back.

2. Your second option is to take the advice of your orthopedic doctor. He or she will either ask you to take pain meds as necessary – *prepare for dangerous spinal fusion surgery with risk of complications* – or ask you to give up your hard-earned money for generic physical therapy treatments, which only give you temporary relief at best.

3. The third option is to try a custom-designed, home-based exercise program which has been specifically created for your scoliosis. With a home exercise-based scoliosis treatment system, you finally can fight your scoliosis and take back control of your life.

Which sounds like the **BEST OPTION** to you?

Remember, waiting longer will only give more opportunity for scoliosis curves to worsen! But, exercise-based scoliosis treatment has been **PROVEN to WORK**.

WHY NOT let it work for **YOU**?

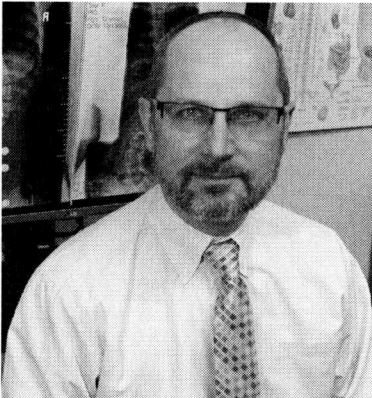

Yours in health,
Dr. Andrew Strauss, BS, DC, MS

P.S. Remember that all severe scoliosis curves have one thing in common; they started out as mild curves and progressively got worse. Do something about your scoliosis N-O-W and reclaim control over your life. I have treated scoliosis curves ranging from mild to severe and patients from age 7 to age 83, but the sooner you start intensive scoliosis treatment, the better the results will be.

So, make that leap of faith today.

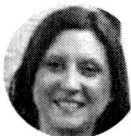

I was unable to find scoliosis treatment anywhere else. Friendly and understanding staff. I was extremely satisfied and would highly recommend it to others needing scoliosis treatment. I would like to say a huge thank you to all the staff and Dr. Strauss from Hudson Valley. You have helped me physically and emotionally. You have also helped me to understand my condition better. I would highly recommend Hudson Valley to others. I believe some people are recommended surgery when there are alternatives that should be explored first.

- Joanna, England

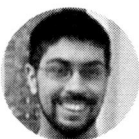

"I'm very happy with Hudson Valley Scoliosis, I like seeing improvement."

– Damon, New Jersey

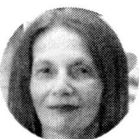

I was searching on the internet for an alternative other than surgery for scoliosis. I was impressed with what I read about Dr. Strauss's method of treatment. Dr. Strauss and the staff were both efficient and personable, and I was treated as an individual not just another body with a problem.

I was given encouragement and hope despite my age and severe degree of curvature and was not just a "foregone conclusion."

I would tell anyone to inquire about Dr. Strauss's method of treatment and to avoid surgery at all costs. Surgery is a very risky procedure and the outcome could be devastating.

- Rose, New Jersey

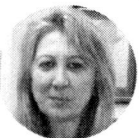

I am satisfied.

- Patrizia, Italy

Very professional, personable, high level of care and genuine concern from staff. Instant feeling of trust with Dr. Strauss, his positive energy and warm vibe.

- Mary, Canada

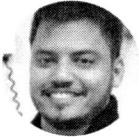

Visit Dr. Strauss, this practice works.

- Ahmed, Trinidad

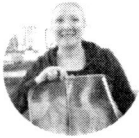

I found the clinic on the internet. I thought the feedback was positive and helpful. I was impressed that I got to speak to Dr. Strauss before coming and my emails with questions were answered promptly and with care. I was very satisfied with the treatment. The office and staff were very efficient, professional, and friendly. All the staff takes time and effort to make sure everything is running correctly and smoothly. Dr. Strauss explains everything and always has time for you. I felt really comfortable and had fun too while having the treatments. Great crowd, great team, great clinic!

- Ursula, Germany

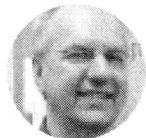

Before I came to you for treatment I was in almost constant pain. My posture was all wrong due to compensating. The compensating created more pain. Now I do my exercises, which you gave me, most days, I rarely suffer from pain and feel like a new man. My posture is good. I constantly think about the right way to stand. Life is good, now!! Thanks Doc.

- John, BC, Canada

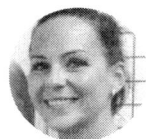

I was referred to Hudson Valley Scoliosis by Dr. "M". Excellent office, pleasant staff, relaxed environment. It was a pleasure to be here. I am completely satisfied. See Dr. Strauss! He is wonderful!

- Diane, New Jersey

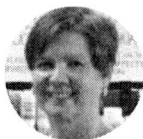

I was referred to Dr. Strauss by my chiropractor. I like the kind and caring treatment by the entire staff. I was very comfortable with the level of experience and kindness of Dr. Strauss. It was important to me that he was affiliated with a research institute such as the CLEAR Method. I was extremely satisfied with the program of care at Hudson Valley Scoliosis Center. It is extremely (and impressively) organized. I can stand straighter and taller than before and I feel great! It has been a positive experience for me!

- Kathleen, New York

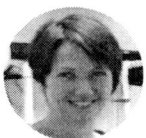

I like Dr. Strauss's thoroughness and that he is so committed to getting an improvement. I am very satisfied. All the staff are very friendly and professional, and everyone treats you with care and consideration. Darleen is a special lady! Definitely try Hudson Valley Scoliosis first--you have nothing to lose.

- Mandy, South Africa

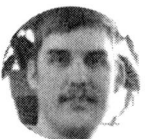

I chose Hudson Valley Scoliosis because of all the good experiences that I heard about and we had a friend that came here. Everyone was very nice and extremely professional and knowledgeable. I noticed a change almost immediately.

- Matthew, Georgia

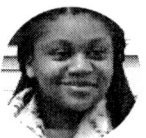

I am really satisfied with the program. I feared that I wouldn't get much results within the 5 days, but I've seen great improvement and wouldn't hesitate to make a revisit.

- Tamilee, Canada

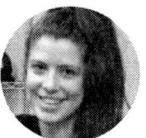

I liked that it was an alternative to bracing. 100 percent satisfied. Try Hudson Valley Scoliosis first you can make improvements to your back without torturing yourself.

- Anna, New Jersey

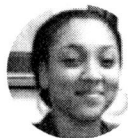

Surgery wasn't an option for us and after doing thorough research Dr. Strauss had all questions answered when I spoke to him and his staff over the phone. I am really satisfied with the care and treatment of the facility because his staff all made me feel at home with very warm hearts. They exceeded my expectations. Dr. Strauss is very detail oriented and treats each of his patients himself. While I was in treatment, I spoke to numerous past and present patients and all said and spoke positive and successful stories. I am very happy with my results.

- Shonda, Trinidad

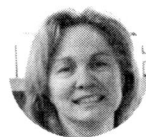

I liked many things about your clinic, but your greatest assets are: the time you spend with every client (you take all the time required to answer questions & solve problems) and the relaxed atmosphere you create here.

Definitely investigate this alternative first. I admit I was skeptical. How could my 50-year-old back "learn new tricks"? But change has occurred.

- Karen, Ohio

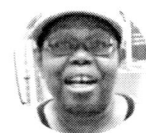

*"I've forgotten about having pain.
I really have."*

Denise, New York

I am a professor of chest medicine and was searching the web for the best center for scoliosis treatment for my daughter. After examining all of the choices, I selected the Hudson Valley Scoliosis Center. What is most important and caught my attention is the highly skillful evaluation and way of practice at the center. The Doctor and staff were very excellent.

- Prof. Dr. S, Egypt (Consultant Pulmonologist)

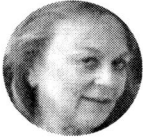

The program here was closest to what I wanted. The center is organized and competent. Reasonable price for the services. would recommend you to anyone.

- Paula, Massachusetts

Since the orthopedic surgeons were pushing for surgery, it only made sense to give this a shot. I am very satisfied with the treatment and feel like it is valuable. Patients debating about this treatment option should give this a shot. What is there to lose? If I had done this earlier, my curve would not have gotten this worse. Waiting is the biggest mistake anyone can do. To anyone debating among treatment options, give this a shot. It can change your life.

- Aiswaria, New York

I am satisfied with the program. I would recommend this approach before bracing or surgery.

- Amanda, Nigeria

Dr. Strauss is a fantastic doctor, very impressed with his knowledge and thorough work. The staff are all very pleasant, welcoming and knowledgeable as well. Great experience overall from the minute we walked in the door.

- Pina, Canada

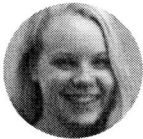

"I am extremely happy with the treatment I have received. Come to Hudson Valley Scoliosis for treatment, because it will make you feel so much better – as it did for me.

Lydia, New Jersey

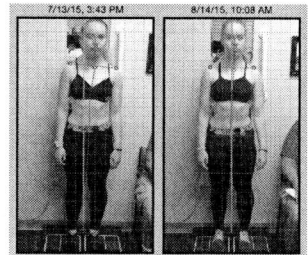

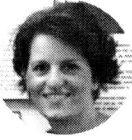

"Very satisfied! Just what I always tell my patients, "EXPLORE CONSERVATIVE, NON-OPERATIVE TREATMENTS FIRST."

Dr. R., Washington, D.C. (Physical Therapist)

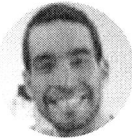

Comprehensive non-surgical spine care center that give patients many options on treating many different health concerns. Very satisfied: very professional and friendly staff. Nice facilities and equipment and treatment is well-supervised and developed. Made my back feel a lot better. Loved my time here! I can't say enough about Dr. Strauss: How knowledgeable and kind of a human being he is. The staff here is awesome: supportive, caring and very professional. Thanks!! Please exhaust every available resource before considering surgery. Many of these treatments are life-changing and will make your quality of life so much better.

- Alfredo, Panama

I like everything about the center. The staff, the hospitality, the care, the concern shown to the patient and family is overwhelming. This place is a great place. Very satisfied.

- Dr. O, Nigeria

FAQs

We understand that you may have questions about the effectiveness of this treatment for your particular situation. Please take a look at our frequently asked questions below. If you don't find the answer to your questions, we would be happy to answer them. Simply call us to learn more about how home exercise-based treatment can improve your specific situation. Dr. Strauss will personally take your call and answer your questions.

"My scoliosis has already progressed significantly. Is it too late for treatment?"

No. While early intervention before the progression of curves is always preferable, we have seen patient after patient reduce their curves and experience relief from their pain and disability using these exercises. We may only be able to modestly straighten your spine, but significant pain control along with life changing postural and cosmetic changes are still very likely.

We understand the pain and helplessness you feel, but there is something you can do about your condition. Don't watch your curves progress for a single day longer than you already have.

"I have a mild curve. Do I qualify for treatment?"

Yes. Patients with a curvature(s) of less than 25 degrees with mild degeneration and low pain levels respond the best to exercise-based programs of care. All severe curves have one thing in common: they all started as mild curves. There is great potential for you to reduce pain and the risk of further progression and even reverse the curve you already have. The best time to treat scoliosis is before progression, severe degeneration or pain.

"I have a severe curve. Do I qualify for treatment?"

Yes. Patients with a curvature(s) of more than 25 degrees require longer treatment because rigidity and compensations have complicated the scoliosis care plan required. While it is always preferable to begin intervention before scoliosis progresses, it is never too late to begin your treatment. Most will see results within weeks.

"Does your office treat all ages?"

Yes. Our youngest patient right now is 7 years old and our oldest is 94. No matter what age or stage you are experiencing, the time to prevent further progression and reduce the risk of pain and disability is now.

"Can I receive treatment if I do not live in the area?"

Yes. We offer special 1-3 week intensive treatment plans that work effectively when combined with at-home exercises. This approach is ideal for out-of-town guests. We have had many patients visit our office from all over the country and the world. Please call us today to arrange your visit. Our helpful staff will assist you with everything you need to know, including:

- Directions

- Accommodations (We have two Hilton hotels next door. They typically offer our patients discounted rates.)

- Travel and US Visa assistance

Don't let location be the only obstacle to receiving the treatment that will change your life forever. Call us today to arrange your customized treatment plan.

"What if it doesn't work?"

What do you have to lose by giving the home exercise-based solution a try? There are:

- No scars

- No drugs (although I do use traditional Chinese herbals)

- No more feeling like there is nothing you can do

"I would like to speak with the doctor directly to decide if this solution is right for me. May I?"

Of course! Our team is awaiting your call. Dr. Strauss will personally respond to your request to discuss your case.

Works Cited

"510(k) Summary - U.S. Food and Drug Administration." 2016. Web. 27 Apr. 2016. https://www.accessdata.fda.gov/cdrh_docs/pdf6/K060043. pdf

"About CLEAR | CLEAR Scoliosis Institute." 2016. Web. 23 Apr. 2016. https://www.clear-institute.org/about/

"Acupuncture | NCCIH." 2015. Web. 23 Apr. 2016. https://nccih.nih.gov/ health/acupuncture

"Adults with Idiopathic Scoliosis Improve Disability ... - Springer." 2016. Web. 11 Apr. 2016. http://link.springer.com/content/pdf/10.1007 per-cent2Fs00586-016-4528-y.pdf

Akazawa, Tsutomu et al. "Corrosion of Spinal Implants Retrieved from Patients with Scoliosis." *Journal of Orthopaedic Science* 10.2 (2005): 200-205. Print.

Allred, CC. "Successful Use of Noninvasive Ventilation in Pregnancy." 2014. Web. 25 Apr. 2016. http://err.ersjournals.com/content/23/131/142.full.pdf

Ambrosio L, Tanner E. Biomaterials for spinal surgery. Amsterdam: Elsevier; 2012.

Beauchamp, Marc et al. "Diurnal Variation of Cobb Angle Measurement in Adolescent Idiopathic Scoliosis." *Spine* 18.12 (1993): 1581-1583. Web. 18 Apr. 2016.

Berdishevsky,H., et al. "Physiotherapy scoliosis-specific exercises – a comprehensive review of seven major schools." *Scoliosis Spinal Disorders.* 2016; 11: 20. https://www.ncbi.nlm.nih.gov/pmc/articles/PMC4973373

Blount WP, Mellencamp D. "The effect of pregnancy on idiopathic scoliosis." —NCBI. 1980. https://www.ncbi.nlm.nih.gov/pubmed/7430194

Burwell, R Geoffrey et al. "Whither the Etiopathogenesis (and Scoliogeny) of Adolescent Idiopathic Scoliosis? Incorporating Presentations on Scoliogeny at the 2012 IRSSD and SRS Meetings." *Scoliosis* 8.1 (2013): 4. Web. 21 Apr. 2016.

Burwell, RG. "Adolescent Idiopathic Scoliosis (AIS), Environment ..." 2011. Web. 25 Apr. 2016. http://scoliosisjournal.biomedcentral.com/articles/10.1186/1748-7161-6-26

Burwell, RG. "Scoliogeny of Adolescent Idiopathic Scoliosis: Inviting ..." 2013. Web. 25 Apr. 2016. http://scoliosisjournal.biomedcentral.com/articles/10.1186/1748-7161-8-8

"Can you be Allergic to Spine Hardware? | Dr. Stefano ..." 2014. Web. 25 Apr. 2016. http://sinicropispine.com/can-allergic-spine-hardware/

Catanzariti, JF. "Visual Deficiency and Scoliosis. - NCBI." 2001. Web. 25 Apr. 2016. http://www.ncbi.nlm.nih.gov/pubmed/11148645

"CDC - Ergonomics and Musculoskeletal Disorders - NIOSH ..." 2003. Web. 20 Apr. 2016. http://www.cdc.gov/niosh/topics/ergonomics/

Charosky S, Guigui P, Blamoutier A, Roussouly P, Chopin D. Complications and risk factors of primary adult scoliosis surgery: a multicenter study of 306 patients. Spine (Phila Pa 1976). 2012;37(8):693–700

Chern JS, Kao CC, Lai PL, Lung CW, Chen WJ. "Severity of spine malalignment on center of pressure progression during level walking in subjects with adolescent idiopathic scoliosis." —NCBI. 2014. https://www.ncbi.nlm.nih.gov/pubmed/25571336

"Chiari Malformation Fact Sheet." 2006. Web. 23 Mar. 2016. http://www.ninds.nih.gov/disorders/chiari/detail_chiari.htm

Chin KR, Furey C, Bohlman HH. "Risk of progression in de novo low-magnitude degenerative lumbar curves: natural history and literature review." *American Journal of Orthopedics.* (Belle Mead NJ). 2009 Aug;38(8):404-9. https://www.ncbi.nlm.nih.gov/pubmed/19809605

"Chiropractic: The Palmer Method (1963) - Chirobase." Web. 27 Apr. 2016. http://www.chirobase.org/05RB/BCC/11a.html

Cho, K, Kim,Y,Shin, S., Suk, S. "Surgical Treatment of Adult Degenerative Scoliosis." *Asian Spine Journal*. 2014 Jun; 8(3): 371–381. https://www.ncbi.nlm.nih.gov/pmc/articles/PMC4068860/

Choudhry MN, Ahmad Z, Verma R (2016) Adolescent idiopathic scoliosis. *Open Orthop J* 10:143–154 https://www.ncbi.nlm.nih.gov/pmc/articles/PMC4897334/

"Classification (King - Lenke) - Harms-Spinesurgery.com." 2007. Web. 27 Apr. 2016. http://harms-spinesurgery.com/src/plugin.php?m=harms.SKO03P

Cobb JR. "Outline for the study of scoliosis." *The American Academy of Orthopedic Surgeons Instructional* Course Lectures. Vol. 5. Ann Arbor, MI: Edwards; 1948.

Cole, D., Ilharreborde, B., Woo, R. (2015) Retrospective Cost Effectiveness Analysis of Implanet Jazz Sublaminar Bands for Surical Treatment of Adolescent Idiopathic Scoliosis. Web. 23 Apr. 2016. http://www.implanet.com/wp-content/themes/theme-implanet/pdf/Health_Advances_Jazz_Cost-Effectiveness.pdf

Dastych, M. "Changes of Selenium, Copper, and Zinc Content in Hair and ..." 2008. Web. 25 Apr. 2016. http://www.ncbi.nlm.nih.gov/pubmed/18404661

Dastych, M. "Idiopathic Scoliosis and Concentrations of Zinc ... - NCBI." 2002. Web. 25 Apr. 2016. http://www.ncbi.nlm.nih.gov/pubmed/12449234

Deckey, Jeffrey E., and David S. Bradford. "Loss of Sagittal Plane Correction after Removal of Spinal Implants." *Spine* 25.19 (2000): 2453-2460. Print.

"Die Skoliose in ihrer Behandlung und Entstehung nach ..." 2013. Web. 20 Apr. 2016. http://www.worldcat.org/title/skoliose-in-ihrer-behandlung-und-entstehung-nach-klinischen-und-experimentellen-studien/oclc/21218666

Dietz, V. "Proprioception and Locomotor Disorders - UFJF." 2002. Web. 25 Apr. 2016. http://www.ufjf.br/especializacaofisioto/files/2013/06/Proprioception-and-locomotor-disorders.pdf

Dobbs, MB. "Prevalence of Neural Axis Abnormalities in Patients with ..." 2002. Web. 26 Apr. 2016. http://www.ncbi.nlm.nih.gov/pubmed/12473713

Drza-Grabiec, J. "Effects of the Sitting Position on the Body Posture of ... - NCBI." 2015. Web. 26 Apr. 2016. http://www.ncbi.nlm.nih.gov/pubmed/24962297

"EMG (Electromyogram) - KidsHealth." 2016. Web. 23 Apr. 2016. http://kidshealth.org/parent/general/sick/emg.html

Fayssoux, RS. "A history of Bracing for Idiopathic Scoliosis in North America." 2010. Web. 20 Apr. 2016. http://www.ncbi.nlm.nih.gov/pubmed/19462214

Frigerio, E. "Metal Sensitivity in Patients with Orthopaedic Implants: a ..." 2011. Web. 26 Apr. 2016. http://www.ncbi.nlm.nih.gov/pubmed/21480913

Gaudreault, N. "Assessment of the Paraspinal Muscles of Subjects Presenting." 2005. Web. 23 Apr. 2016. http://bmcmusculoskeletdisord.biomedcentral.com/articles/10.1186/1471-2474-6-14

"Gene CHD7 linked with Scoliosis [Archive] - National ..." 2009. Web.15 Apr. 2016. http://www.scoliosis.org/forum/archive/index.php/t-8938.html

"Genetic Scoliosis Research - Texas Scottish Rite Hospital ..." 2013. Web.15 Apr. 2016. http://www.tsrhc.org/genetic-scoliosis-research

Guo, J. "A Prospective Randomized Controlled Study on the Treatment ..." 2014. Web. 26 Apr. 2016. http://link.springer.com/article/10.1007 percent2Fs00586-013-3146-1

Hahn, Frederik, Reinhard Zbinden, and Kan Min. "Late Implant Infections Caused by Propionibacterium Acnes in Scoliosis Surgery." *European Spine Journal* 14.8 (2005): 783-788. Print.

Hawes, M.C. (2002). *Scoliosis and the Human Spine.* Tucson, Arizona: West Press. Print.

Herman R, Mixon J, Fisher A, Maulucci R, Stuyck J. "Idiopathic scoliosis and the central nervous system: a motor control problem. The Harrington lecture, 1983. Scoliosis Research Society." *Spine* (Phila Pa 1976). 1985 Jan-Feb; 10(1):1-14

"Holistic Medicine: What It Is, Treatments ... - WebMD." 2012. Web. 27 Apr. 2016. http://www.webmd.com/balance/guide/what-is-holistic-medicine

"Homeopathy - Wikipedia, the Free Encyclopedia." 2011. Web. 27 Apr. 2016. https://en.wikipedia.org/wiki/Homeopathy

Huh, S. "Cardiopulmonary Function and Scoliosis Severity in ... - NCBI." 2015. Web. 26 Apr. 2016. http://www.ncbi.nlm.nih.gov/pmc/articles/PMC4510355/

"Index of Paper_pdf - Osteopathic Research Web." 2012. Web. 20 Apr. 2016. http://www.osteopathic-research.com/paper_pdf/

"Infantile Scoliosis - Medscape Reference." Web. 23 Mar. 2016. http://emedicine.medscape.com/article/1259899-overview

"Introduction to Vinyasa Flow Yoga - Health." 2016. Web. 27 Apr. 2016. https://www.verywell.com/introduction-to-vinyasa-flow-yoga-3566892

Isaacs, RE, Hyde, J., Goodrich, J.A; Rodgers, WB, Phillips, F. "A Prospective, Nonrandomized, Multicenter Evaluation of Extreme Lateral Interbody Fusion for the Treatment of Adult Degenerative Scoliosis: Perioperative Outcomes and Complications." Spine: Dec., 2010 35(26S). S322-S330. https://journals.lww.com/spinejournal/Abstract/2010/12151/A_Prospective,_Nonrandomized,_Multicenter.8.aspx

Jiang J, Meng Y, Jin X, Zhang C, Zhao J, Wang C, Gao R, Zhou X. "Volumetric and fatty infiltration imbalance of deep paravertebral muscles in adolescent idiopathic scoliosis." *Med Sci Monit.* 2017;23:2089–2095.

Ji, X et al. "Change of Selenium in Environment and Risk of Adolescent Idiopathic Scoliosis: a Retrospective Cohort Study." *Eur Rev Med Pharmacol Sci* 17.18 (2013): 2499-503. Web. 21 Apr. 2016.

Jokar, M. "Epidemiology of Vasculitides in Khorasan Province, Iran." 2015. Web. 26 Apr. 2016. http://www.ncbi.nlm.nih.gov/pmc/articles/PMC4487463/

Journal of Maternity Fetal and Neonatal Medicine 2012 Jun;25(6):631-41.

Jull, GA. "Motor Control Problems in Patients with Spinal Pain: a New ..." 2000. Web. 26 Apr. 2016. http://www.ncbi.nlm.nih.gov/pubmed/10714539

"Khan Kinetic Treatment." 2015. Web. 27 Apr. 2016. http://www.moh.gov.my/attachments/7489.pdf

Kilshaw M, Baker RP, Gardner R, Charosky S, Harding I. "Abnormalities of the lumbar spine in the coronal plane on plain abdominal radiographs." *European Spine Journal.* 2011 Mar;20(3):429-33. https://www.ncbi.nlm.nih.gov/pubmed/21069544

Kim, HD. "Electron Microprobe Analysis and Tissue Reaction ... - NCBI." 2007. Web. 26 Apr. 2016. http://www.ncbi.nlm.nih.gov/pmc/articles/PMC2857498/

Kluba T, Dikmenli G, Dietz K, Giehl JP, Niemeyer T. "Comparison of surgical and conservative treatment for degenerative lumbar scoliosis." *Archives of Orthopedic Trauma Surgery.* 2009 Jan;129(1):1-5. https://www.ncbi.nlm.nih.gov/pubmed/18560848

Ko DY, Lee HS. "The Changes of COP and Foot Pressure after One Hour's Walking Wearing High-heeled and Flat Shoes." *Journal of Physical Therapy Science.* 2013 Oct;25(10):1309-12. https://www.ncbi.nlm.nih.gov/pubmed/24259782

Kotwal, S, Pumberger, M., Hughes, A., Girardi, F. "Degenerative Scoliosis: A Review." *HSS Journal* (2011) 7: 257. https://doi.org/10.1007/s11420-011-9204-5.

Knott, Patrick et al. "SOSORT 2012 Consensus paper: Reducing X-ray Exposure in Pediatric Patients with Scoliosis." *Scoliosis* 9.1 (2014): 1. Web. 21 Apr. 2016.

Kruse, LM. "Polygenic Threshold Model with Sex Dimorphism in ... - NCBI." 2012. Web. 26 Apr. 2016. http://www.ncbi.nlm.nih.gov/pubmed/22992817

Kulis, Aleksandra et al. "Participation of Sex Hormones in Multifactorial Pathogenesis of Adolescent Idiopathic Scoliosis." *International Orthopaedics* 39.6 (2015): 1227-1236. Web. 19 Apr. 2016.

Lantz, Charles A, and Jasper Chen. "Effect of Chiropractic Intervention on Small Scoliotic Curves in Younger Subjects: a Time-Series Cohort Design." *Journal of Manipulative and Physiological Therapeutics* 24.6 (2001): 385-393. Print.

"Lenke Classification System for Scoliosis | Lawrence Lenke ..." 2012. Web. 24 Mar. 2016. http://spinal-deformity-surgeon.com/a-leader-in-spinal-deformity/lenke-classification-system-for-scoliosis/

Linder M, Saltzman CL. "A history of medical scientists on high heels." *International Journal of Health Services.* 1998;28(2):2012 http://ir.uiowa.edu/cgi/viewcontent.cgi?article=1074&context=law_pubs

"Lumbar Fusion | University of Maryland Medical Center." Web. 26 Apr. 2016. http://umm.edu/programs/spine/health/guides/lumbar-fusion

Mahmood, SS. "The Framingham Heart Study and the Epidemiology ... - NCBI." 2014. Web. 25 Apr. 2016. http://www.ncbi.nlm.nih.gov/pmc/articles/PMC4159698/

Marty-Poumarat et.al. (Spine 2007) Natural History of Progressive Adult Scoliosis.

McWilliams DF, Muthuri S, Muir KR, Maciewicz RA, Zhang W, Doherty M. "Self-reported adult footwear and the risks of lower limb osteoarthritis: the GOAL case control study." *BMC Musculoskeletal Disorders.* 2014 Sep 20;15:308. http://www.ncbi.nlm.nih.gov/pubmed/25240981

Mika A, Oleksy L, Mika P, Marchewka A, Clark BC. "The effect of walking in high- and low-heeled shoes on erector spinae activity and pelvis kinematics during gait." *American Journal of Physical and Medical Rehabilitation.* 2012 May;91(5):425-34. https://www.ncbi.nlm.nih.gov/pubmed/22311060

Modi, HN. "Scoliosis and Spinal Disorders | Pre-publication history ..." 2009. Web. 26 Apr. 2016. http://www.scoliosisjournal.com/content/4/1/11/prepub

Morningstar, MW. "Scoliosis Treatment Using a Combination of Manipulative and ..." 2004. Web. 26 Apr. 2016. http://bmcmusculoskeletdisord.biomedcentral.com/articles/10.1186/1471-2474-5-32

National Scoliosis Foundation. "Instrumentation Systems For Scoliosis Surgery". National Scoliosis Foundation. Retrieved February 11, 2010.

Negrini, S., et al. "2016 SOSORT guidelines: orthopaedic and rehabilitation treatment of idiopathic scoliosis during growth." *Scoliosis and Spinal Disorders.* 2018;13:3. https://scoliosisjournal.biomedcentral.com/articles/10.1186/s13013-017-0145-8

Negrini, A. "Scoliosis-Specific Exercises can Reduce the Progression of ..." 2015. Web. 26 Apr. 2016. http://www.ncbi.nlm.nih.gov/pmc/articles/PMC4537533/

Niesluchowski, W. "The Potential Role of Brain Asymmetry in the Development of ..." 1999. Web. 25 Apr. 2016. http://www.ncbi.nlm.nih.gov/pubmed/10543585

Orvomaa, E. "Pregnancy and Delivery in Patients Operated by the ... - NCBI." 1997. Web. 26 Apr. 2016. http://www.ncbi.nlm.nih.gov/pubmed/9391799

Pace, Nicola, Leonardo Ricci, and Stefano Negrini. "A Comparison Approach to Explain Risks Related to X-ray Imaging for Scoliosis, 2012 SOSORT award winner." *Scoliosis* 8.11 (2013): 7161-8. Web.19 Apr. 2016.

Page, P. "Cervicogenic Headaches: an Evidence-Led Approach ... - NCBI." 2011.Web. 26 Apr. 2016. http://www.ncbi.nlm.nih.gov/pubmed/22034615

Palazzo, C., et al. "Effects of Bracing in Adult With Scoliosis: A Retrospective Study." *Archives of Physical Medicine and Rehabilitation.* January 2017Volume 98, Issue 1, Pages 187–190

"Patient Controlled Analgesia (PCA) Pumps: The Basics." 2015. Web. 25 Apr. 2016. http://www.ppahs.org/2012/05/patient-controlled-analgesia-pca-pumps-the-basics/

Pehrsson,K, Bake,B, Larsson, S, Nachemson, A. "Lung function in adult idiopathic scoliosis: a 20 year follow up." —NCBI. 1991. https://www.ncbi.nlm.nih.gov/pmc/articles/PMC463231/

"Questions and Answers about Scoliosis in Children and ..." 2008. Web. 27 Apr. 2016. http://www.niams.nih.gov/Health_Info/Scoliosis/

Renshaw, T. S. "The Role of Harrington Instrumentation and Posterior Spine Fusion in the Management of Adolescent Idiopathic Scoliosis." *The Orthopedic Clinics of North America* 19.2 (1988): 257-267. Print.

Reynolds, RA. "Postoperative Pain Management after Spinal Fusion Surgery ..." 2013. Web. 26 Apr. 2016. http://www.ncbi.nlm.nih.gov/pubmed/24436846

Rullander, AC. "Young People's Experiences with Scoliosis Surgery: a Survey ..." 2013. Web. 26 Apr. 2016. http://www.ncbi.nlm.nih.gov/pubmed/24247313

Rullander, Anna-Clara et al. "Young People's Experiences with Scoliosis Surgery: a Survey of Pain, Nausea, and Global Satisfaction." *Orthopaedic Nursing* 32.6 (2013): 327-333. Print.

Sadat-Ali M, Al-Othman A, Bubshait D, Al-Dakheel D. "Does scoliosis causes low bone mass? A comparative study between siblings." *European Spine Journal.* 2008 Jul;17(7):944–947. https://www.ncbi.nlm.nih.gov/pmc/articles/PMC2443267/

Sahay, M. "Rickets – Vitamin D Deficiency and Dependency - NCBI." 2012. Web. 26 Apr. 2016. http://www.ncbi.nlm.nih.gov/pmc/articles/PMC3313732/

Saunders, Travis J, Jean-Philippe Chaput, and Mark S Tremblay. "Sedentary Behaviour as an Emerging Risk Factor for Cardiometabolic Diseases in Children and Youth." *Canadian Journal of Diabetes* 38.1 (2014): 53-61. Print.

Schimmel, JJP. "Adolescent Idiopathic Scoliosis and Spinal Fusion do not Substantially ..." 2015. Web. 26 Apr. 2016. http://www.ncbi.nlm.nih.gov/pmc/articles/PMC4459442/

Schroeder, J.,Dettori,JR, Ecker,E, and Kaplan, L." Does pregnancy increase curve progression in women with scoliosis treated without surgery?" *Evidence-Based Spine-Care Journal.* 2011 Aug; 2(3): 43–50. https://www.ncbi.nlm.nih.gov/pmc/articles/PMC3604750/

"Scoliosis – Disease Index, Musculo-Skeletal – Hpathy.com." 2011. Web. 27 Apr. 2016. http://hpathy.com/cause-symptoms-treatment/scoliosis/

"Scoliosis | Wunderkammer." 2012. Web. 20 Apr. 2016. http://wunderkammer.ki.se/images/scoliosis

"Scoliosis and Bach flowers – Alternative ..." 2007. Web. 27 Apr. 2016. http://scoliosis.homestead.com/bachflowers.html

"Scoliosis Research Society." 2015. Web. 25 Apr. 2016. https://www.srs.org/chinese_sim/patient_and_family/the_aging_spine/pseudarthrosis.htm

"Scoliosis Surgery: Things to Consider-OrthoInfo - AAOS." 2011. Web. 25 Apr. 2016. http://orthoinfo.aaos.org/topic.cfm?topic=A00641

Shang, X. "Metal Hypersensitivity in Patient with Posterior Lumbar Spine ..." 2014. Web. 25 Apr. 2016. http://bmcmusculoskeletdisord.biomed-central.com/articles/10.1186/1471-2474-15-314

Shang, Xianping et al. "Metal Hypersensitivity in Patient with Posterior Lumbar Spine Fusion: a Case Report and its Literature Review." *BMC Musculoskeletal Disorders* 15.1 (2014): 314. Print.

Shridharani, S.,Munroe, B., Hood, K. "Complications in adult degenerative scoliosis surgery." *Seminars in Spine Surgery.* 29(2). June 2017. 118-122.

Siegel, JA. "The Birth of the Illegitimate Linear No-Threshold Model: An ..." 2015. Web. 26 Apr. 2016. http://www.ncbi.nlm.nih.gov/pubmed/26535990

Smith JS, Shaffrey CI, Kuntz CT et al. Classification systems for adolescent and adult scoliosis. *Neurosugery.* 2008;63 (3 Suppl):16-24.

"Spinal Fusion: MedlinePlus Medical Encyclopedia." 2006. Web. 26 Apr. 2016. https://www.nlm.nih.gov/medlineplus/ency/article/002968.htm

"SpineCor Dynamic Corrective Brace." 2013. Web. 22 Apr. 2016. http://www.spinecor.com/ForProfessionals/SpineCorDynamicCorrective-Brace.aspx

Strauss, Andrew J., and Charlie Changli Xue. "Acupuncture for Chronic Non-Specific Low Back Pain: A Case Series Study." *Chinese Journal of Integrated Traditional and Western Medicine* 7.3 (2001): 190-194. Print.

Tan, Gabriel et al. "Efficacy of Selected Complementary and Alternative Medicine Interventions for Chronic Pain." *Journal of Rehabilitation Research and Development* 44.2 (2007): 195. Print.

"The History of Lumbar Spine Stabilization." 2005. Web. 26 Apr. 2016. http://www.burtonreport.com/infspine/SurgStabilSpineHistory.htm

"The Schroth Method – Exercises for Scoliosis." 2007. Web. 27 Apr. 2016. http://www.schrothmethod.com/

Thyssen, Jacob Pontoppidan et al. "The Association Between Metal Allergy, Total Hip Arthroplasty, and Revision: A Case-Control Study." *Acta Orthopaedica* 80.6 (2009): 646-652. Print.

Timgren, J. "Reversible Pelvic Asymmetry: an Overlooked ... – NCBI." 2006. Web. 26 Apr. 2016. http://www.ncbi.nlm.nih.gov/pubmed/16949945

Titchenal MR, Asay JL, Favre J, Andriacchi TP, Chu CR." Effects of high heel wear and increased weight on the khttps://www.ncbi.nlm.nih.gov/pubmed/25532875nee during walking." *Journal of Orthopedic Research.* 2015 Mar;33(3):405-11.

Tsiligiannis, T. "Pulmonary Function in Children with Idiopathic Scoliosis | Scoliosis and ..." 2012. Web. 26 Apr. 2016. http://scoliosisjournal.biomedcentral.com/articles/10.1186/1748-7161-7-7

Tsiligiannis, Theofanis, and Theodoros Grivas. "Pulmonary Function in Children with Idiopathic Scoliosis." *Scoliosis* 7.1 (2012): 7. Web. 22 Apr. 2016.

Vasiliadis, ES. "Historical Overview of Spinal Deformities in Ancient Greece ..." 2009. Web. 26 Apr. 2016. http://scoliosisjournal.biomedcentral.com/articles/10.1186/1748-7161-4-6

Warren, Michelle P., Gunn, JB, Hamilton, LH, Warren, LF, and Hamilton, WG. (May 1986). Scoliosis and fractures in young ballet dancers. *New England Journal of Medicine.* 314, 1348-1353. doi: 10.1056/NEJM 198605223142104. Web. 1 May 2016. http://www.nejm.org/doi/pdf/10.1056/nejm198605223142104

Weiner, MF. "Abstract – Nature Publishing Group." 2009. Web. 26 Apr. 2016. http://www.nature.com/sc/journal/v47/n6/abs/sc200919a.html

Weinstein, SL. "Effects of Bracing in Adolescents with Idiopathic ... – NCBI." 2013. Web. 20 Apr. 2016. http://www.ncbi.nlm.nih.gov/pmc/articles/PMC3913566/

Weinstein, SL. "Health and Function of Patients with Untreated ... – NCBI." 2003. Web. 26 Apr. 2016. http://www.ncbi.nlm.nih.gov/pubmed/12578488

Weinstein, SL. "PubMed – NCBI." 2008. Web. 26 Apr. 2016. http://www.ncbi.nlm.nih.gov/pubmed/18456103

Weiss, Hans-Rudolf, and Deborah Goodall. "Rate of Complications in Scoliosis Surgery – a Systematic Review of the PubMed Literature." *Scoliosis* 3.1 (2008): 1. Web. 22 Apr. 2016.

Weiss, HR, and HR Weiss. "Rate of Complications in Scoliosis Surgery – a Systematic... – NCBI." 2008. Web. 26 Apr. 2016. http://www.ncbi.nlm.nih.gov/pmc/articles/PMC2525632/

Weiss HR, Moramarco M, Moramarco K. "Risks and long-term complications of adolescent idiopathic scoliosis surgery versus non-surgical and natural history outcomes." *Hard Tissue* 2013 Apr 30;2(3):27.

Weiss, HR. "Acupuncture in the Treatment of Scoliosis – a Single Blind ..." 2008. Web. 26 Apr. 2016. http://scoliosisjournal.biomedcentral.com/articles/10.1186/1748-7161-3-4

Weiss, HR. "Adolescent Idiopathic Scoliosis – to Operate or Not? A ... – NCBI." 2008. Web. 26 Apr. 2016. http://www.ncbi.nlm.nih.gov/pmc/articles/PMC2572584/

"What Are the Treatments for Mild Scoliosis? | eHow." 2009. Web. 27 Apr. 2016.http://www.ehow.com/facts_5006530_what-treatments-mild-scoliosis.html

Wick, JM. "Infantile and Juvenile Scoliosis: The Crooked Path to ..." 2009. Web. 25 Apr. 2016. http://www.aornjournal.org/article/S0001-2092(09)00551-1/abstract

Worthington, V. "Nutrition as an Environmental Factor in the Etiology of ... – NCBI."1993. Web. 26 Apr. 2016. http://www.ncbi.nlm.nih.gov/pubmed/8492060

Xin-Feng Li, Hai Li, Zu-De Liu, Li-Yang Dai. "Low bone mineral sta-
tus in adolescent idiopathic scoliosis. " *European Spine Journal.* 2008
Nov;17(11):1431–1440.   https://www.ncbi.nlm.nih.gov/pmc/articles/
PMC2583185/

Zabjek, KF. "Acute Postural Adaptations Induced by a Shoe Lift in... –
NCBI." 2001. Web. 19 Apr. 2016. http://www.ncbi.nlm.nih.gov/pu-
bmed/11345630